PREFACE

This is volume three of a four-volume series. The aim is to test diagnostic skills over a wide range of clinical problems. Questions which may feature in examinations or in clinical practice are posed in an attempt to stimulate the undergraduate or postgraduate reader to undertake further reading.

The pictures in this new series have been selected from the clinical slide library in the Department of Medical Illustration, University of Aberdeen. The books have been produced against a background of experience gained over the last 10 years in the compilation for local use of over 2,000 self-assessment examples. The local exercise was coordinated through the Medical Learning Resources Group of the Faculty of Medicine, University of Aberdeen, in collaboration with many of the clinicians in the Aberdeen Teaching Hospitals.

We hope that the books will be of interest to all who are committed to their own continuing medical education. We would welcome comment on individual questions and answers.

GSJC, MJJ, RAM, JCP, HMAT.

Although numbering is sequential, each volume in the series is unique, containing a balanced selection of diagnostic examples, and thus may be used independently.

ACKNOWLEDGEMENTS

We wish to acknowledge the invaluable contribution of Dr Anthony Hedley, now Professor of Community Medicine, University of Glasgow, who was the instigator of the self-assessment programme on which these books are based. We would also like to acknowledge the cooperation of all patients, secretarial and technical staff, in particular the staff of the Department of Medical Illustration, who have contributed in one way or another to the preparation of these volumes, and Mrs Margaret Doverty who typed the manuscript.

We would particularly like to thank the following colleagues for contributing material for the books:

Dr D R Abramovich, Mr A Adam, Mr A K Ah-See, Dr D J G Bain, Dr L S Bain, Dr K Bartlett, Dr A P Bayliss, Dr B Bennett, Miss F M Bennett, Dr P Best, Dr P D Bewsher, Mr C Birchall, Mr C T Blaiklock, Dr L J Borthwick, Mr P L Brunnen, Dr P W Brunt, Dr J Calder, Professor A G M Campbell, Dr B Carrie, Dr P Carter, Dr G R D Catto, Mr R B Chesney, Dr N Clark, Mr P B Clarke, Mr A I Davidson, Dr R J L Davidson, Dr A A Dawson, Mr W B M Donaldson, Professor A S Douglas, Dr A W Downie, Dr C J Eastmond, Mr J Engeset, Dr N Edward, Dr J K Finlayson, Dr J R S Finnie, Mr A V Foote, Dr N G Fraser, Mr R J A Fraser, Dr J A R Friend, Dr D B Galloway, Mr J M C Gibson, Dr D Hadley, Dr J E C Hern, Dr A W Hutcheon, Dr T A Jeffers, Dr A W Johnston, Mr P F Jones, Dr A C F Kenmure, Mr I R Kernohan, Dr A S M Khir, Mr J Kyle, Dr J S Legge, Mr McFadzean, Dr E McKay, Mr J McLauchlan, Mr K A McLay, Professor M MacLeod, Dr R A Main, Mr Mather, Mr N A Matheson, Mr J D B Miller, Mr S S Miller, Mr K L G Mills, Dr N A G Mowat, Mr I F K Muir, Dr L E Murchison, Mr W J Newlands, Mr J G Page, Professor R Postlethwaite, Dr J M Rawles, Mr P K Ray, Mr C R W Rayner, Professor A M Rennie, Mr A G R Rennie, Dr J A N Rennie, Dr O J Robb, Dr H S Ross, Dr G Russell, Dr D S Short, Dr P J Smail, Dr C C Smith, Professor G Smith, Dr L Stankler, Mr J H Steyn, Professor J M Stowers, Dr G H Swapp, Mr J Wallace, Professor W Walker, Dr S J Watt, Dr J Weir, Dr J Webster, Dr M I White, Dr F W Wigzell, Dr M J Williams, Mr L C Wills, Dr L A Wilson, Mr H A Young.

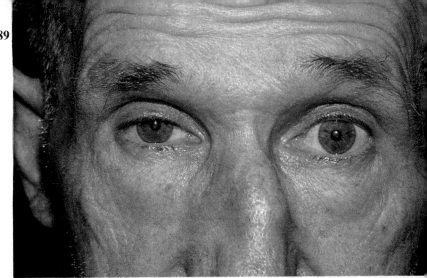

389 and 390

a What neurological
   abnormalities are seen
   in this patient's
   i)   eyes?
   ii) tongue?
b Suggest three possible
   diagnoses.

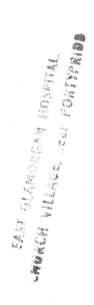

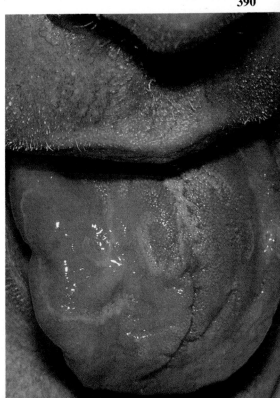

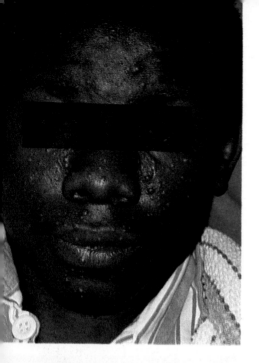

391

391 and 392

a From what condition does this man suffer?

b What principal radiological abnormalities are seen?

c Is any skin test of diagnostic value?

d Which animal is the reservoir of infection?

392

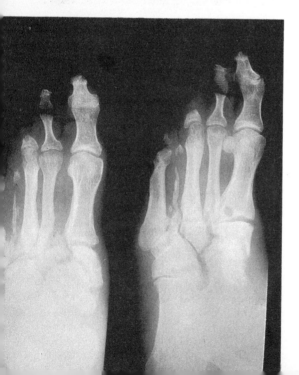

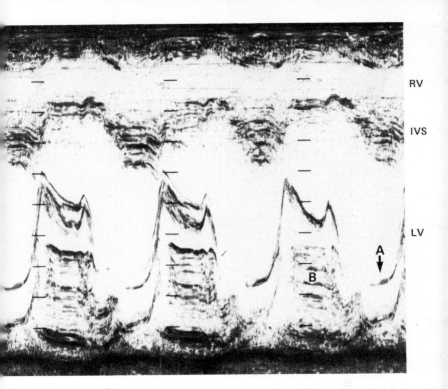

RV

IVS

LV

393 M-mode echocardiogram through the mitral valve
  RV — right ventricle
  LV — left ventricle
  IVS — inter-ventricular septum
  This M-mode echocardiogram is from a twenty-four year old female
  patient who complains of chest pain and palpitations. Praecordial
  auscultation reveals two abnormalities.
  a What are the features marked 'A' and 'B'?
  b What is the diagnosis?
  c What are the typical auscultatory findings in this condition?

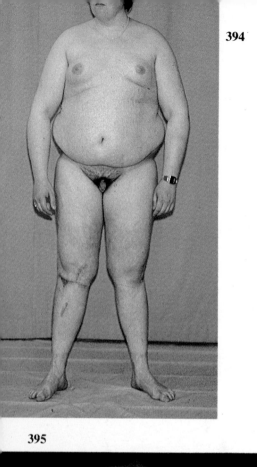

394

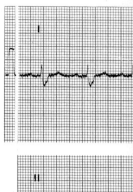

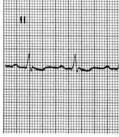

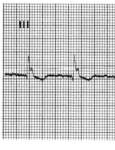

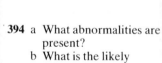

395

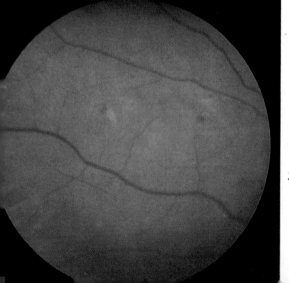

394 a What abnormalities are present?
b What is the likely cause?

395 This is the fundus of a forty-two year old woman with recurrent urinary tract infection.
What is demonstrated?

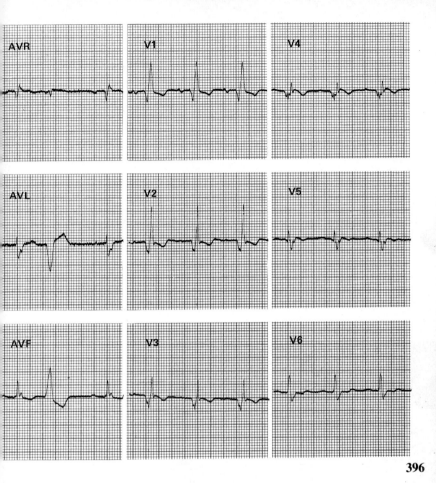

396

396 This man had a normal electrocardiogram five years ago.
   a What abnormalities are present?
   b Is the conduction abnormality of significance?
   c What is the likely cause of the electrical changes?

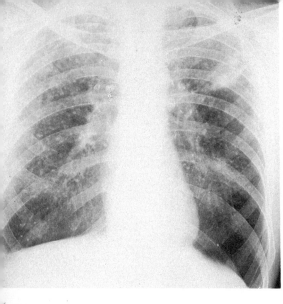

397 This is the chest x-ray of a granite polisher. It was taken at a routine medical examination.
  a Describe the radiological abnormalities.
  b What is the diagnosis?
  c Does this man have an increased risk of
    i) bronchial carcinoma?
    ii) tuberculosis?

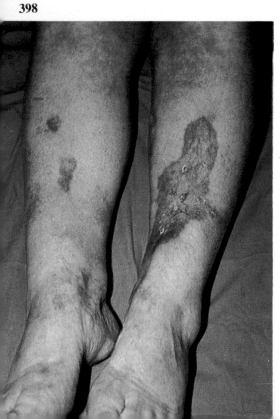

398 This forty-five year old obese female has been aware of gradually enlarging plaques on her shins for several months. She has no other symptoms.
  a Of what condition is this appearance typical?
  b Which metabolic disorder is likely to be present?
  c How does the progress of this disorder relate to the severity of the skin lesions?

399

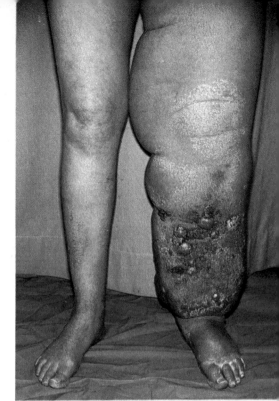

399 a What descriptive name is given to the appearance of this patient's left leg?
   b What is the most common infective cause of this disorder?
   c What abnormality would be expected on inguinal lymph node biopsy?

400 This patient complains of increasing dysphagia with regurgitation of foodstuffs either spontaneously, with changes in position, or with neck massage.
   a What abnormality is seen on barium swallow?
   b Give three pulmonary complications of this disorder.
   c What is the principal hazard of endoscopy in this condition?

400

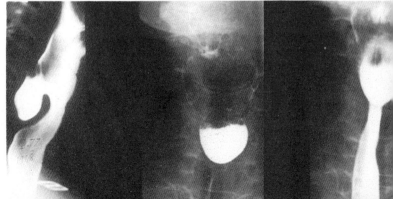

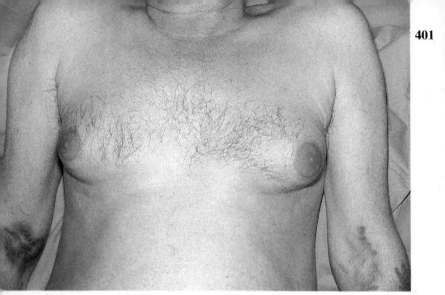

401 This patient is mildly jaundiced.
a What two abnormalities are seen?
b What is the most likely diagnosis?

402

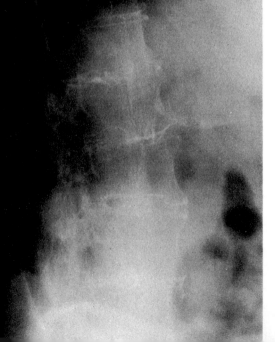

402 What causes this patient's voided urine to darken on standing?

403

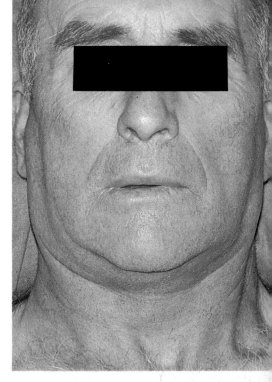

403 This patient has mild conjugated hyperbilirubinaemia.
  a What abnormality is shown?
  b What is the most likely diagnosis?
  c What specific drug treatment may be indicated?

404 This patient was found unconscious.
  a What is the likely cause of her coma?
  b What changes in therapy may improve the abnormality shown?

404

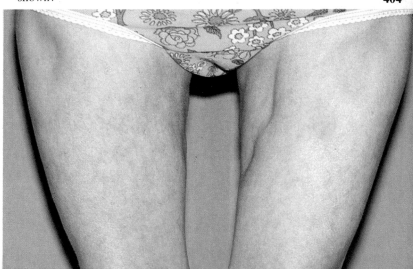

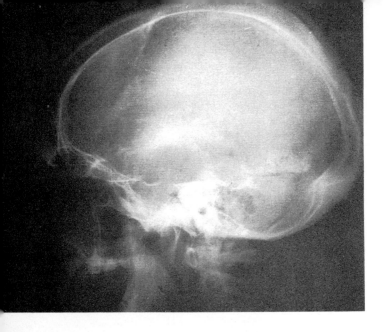

405 and 406 This mentally handicapped child was referred for
   investigation of epilepsy. An abnormality in biochemical screening led
   to closer examination of the child's hands, and to the x-rays shown.
   a What abnormalities are seen in the x-rays of:
      i) skull?
      ii) hands?
   b What unusual diagnosis do these suggest?
   c How may this diagnosis be established biochemically?

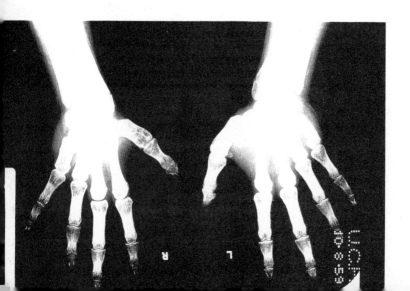

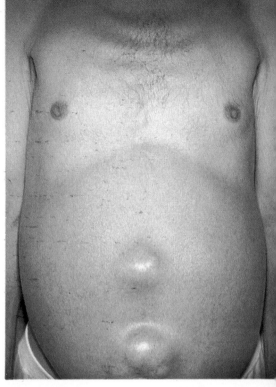

407 This patient presented with abdominal swelling and weight loss. A low grade fever was present and neither liver nor spleen were palpable. Paracentesis produced fluid with a protein content of 40 g/l, glucose 1.9 mmol/l and normal amylase. Cytology showed mesothelial cells and lymphocytes. Gram stain was negative.
   a What is the likely diagnosis?
   b What further investigations are indicated?

408 This Haitian patient gives a four month history of failing central vision in the left eye. For six weeks he has noticed clumsiness of the right hand and now has established pyramidal signs on the right side. He has generalised non-tender lymphadenopathy and a low grade fever.
   a What fundal abnormality is seen?
   b What is the likely cause?
   c How does this relate to the neurological findings?
   d What underlying disorder should be considered?

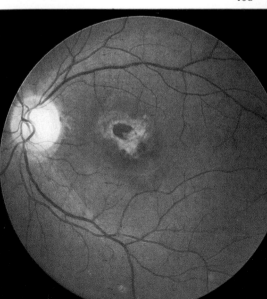

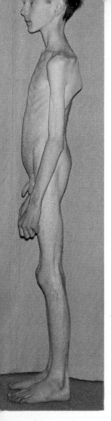

409 During in-patient
   assessment of short
   stature and failure to gain
   weight this ten year old
   boy was found to have
   subnormal responses to
   oral D-xylose and butter
   fat tests. He has no
   abdominal symptoms and
   is otherwise well.
   a What is the most likely
      diagnosis?
   b Which
      histocompatibility
      antigens are more
      common in patients
      with this condition than
      in the general
      population?

410

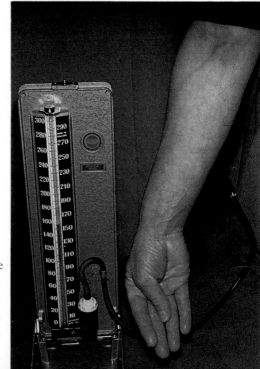

410 a What physical sign is
        illustrated here?
    b What is the significance
       of this positive test?
    c Suggest four
       biochemical
       abnormalities that may
       cause this condition.

411

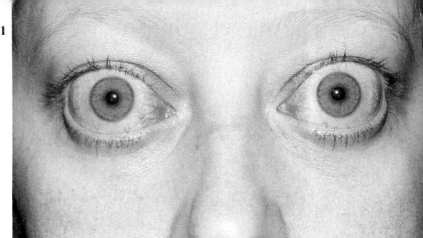

411 a What abnormalities are
     shown here?
   b What is the diagnosis?
   c State two serious ocular
     complications of this
     disorder.
   d What treatment would
     you recommend?

412

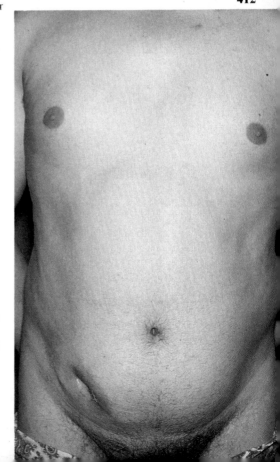

412 Two months ago this
    patient presented with
    symptoms and signs
    suggestive of acute
    appendicitis. At
    operation a normal
    appendix was removed.
   a What abnormality can
     now be seen at the site
     of the appendicectomy
     scar?
   b What is the underlying
     diagnosis?
   c What is likely to have
     been the cause of his
     'acute abdomen'?

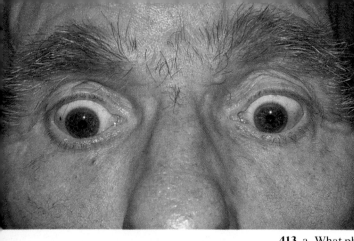

413 a What physical sign is
being demonstrated?
b State the likely
underlying disorder.
c What other ocular signs
of this condition may
be observed or
demonstrated?

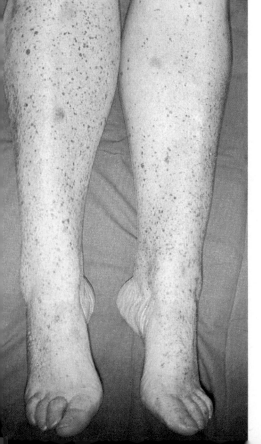

414 This eighteen year old
complained of epistaxis,
menorrhagia, and a rash
on her legs. Blood count
was normal apart from a
platelet count of 10 x
$10^9/1$.
a What is the most likely
diagnosis?
b What would bone
marrow examination
show in this condition?
c What other conditions
should be considered?

415

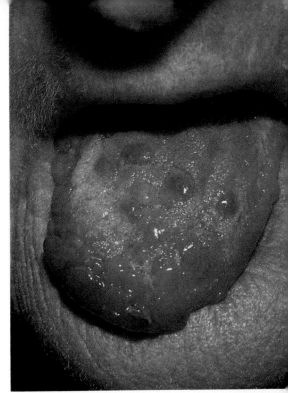

415 This man with nephrotic syndrome complains that his tongue is becoming larger.
a Why?
b How is the diagnosis established?

416

416 What are the pulmonary causes of this abnormality?

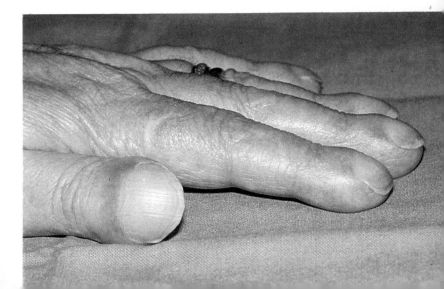

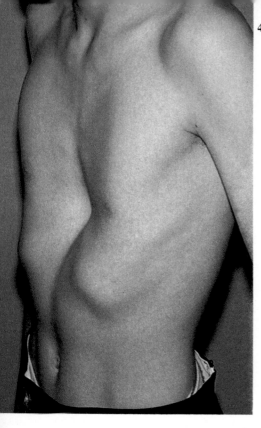

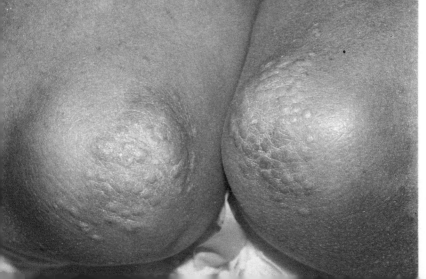

417 Is this boy likely to
develop ventilatory
failure?
What would you expect
pulmonary function
testing to show?

418 This forty-three year old
white woman has
developed severe angina
pectoris.
a What abnormality is
shown?
b What is the likely
diagnosis?
c How is the diagnosis
confirmed?
d What therapeutic
measures may be
indicated?

418

419

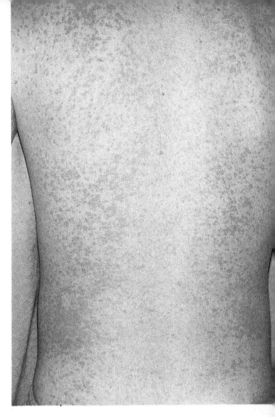

419 This young man was
prescribed ampicillin for a
sore throat.
  a Which organism is most
    likely to have caused
    his sore throat?
  b Which other conditions
    increase the likelihood
    of similar ampicillin
    rashes?
  c Can the patient be
    given penicillin in
    future?

420 This seventy-five year old
man developed increasing
confusion, clumsiness and
incontinence over a five
week period.
  a What is the diagnosis?
  b Which factors are
    thought to be
    important in the
    development of this
    condition?

420

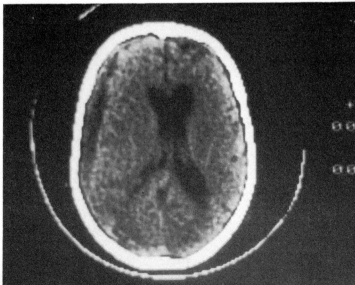

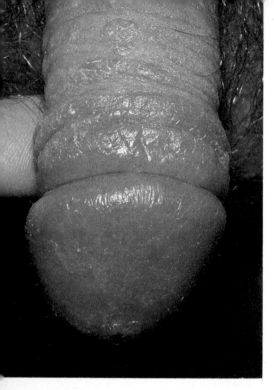

421

421 and 422 This patient
complains of low back
stiffness, worst after
periods of rest, and has
experienced sciatic pains
in both buttocks and
upper legs.
a What principal
abnormality is seen on
pelvic x-ray?
b What abnormality is
seen on the penis?
c What is the diagnosis?
d What is the likelihood
that this patient is HLA
B27 positive?

422

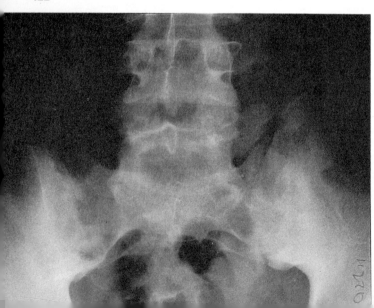

423

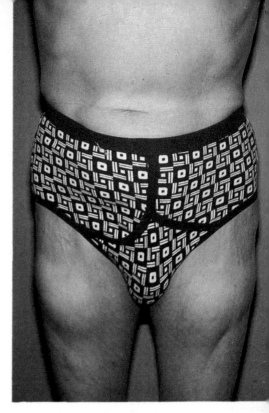

423 This patient with type I diabetes has noticed these lumps on his thighs.
- a What is the nature of the lumps?
- b Explain the underlying pathogenesis of these lesions.
- c What advice would you give this patient?

424 This patient complains of frequent headaches.
- a What diagnosis is suggested by the appearance of his hands?
- b List two tests which are necessary to confirm the diagnosis.

424

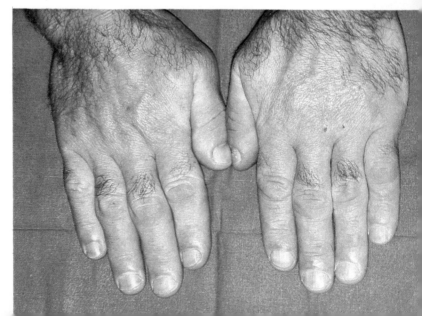

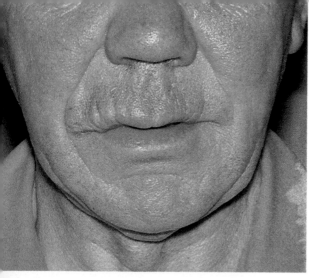

425

425 and 426 These conditions share a common aetiology.
    a What radiological abnormality is present?
    b What name is given to the appearance of the mouth?
    c What is the cause?

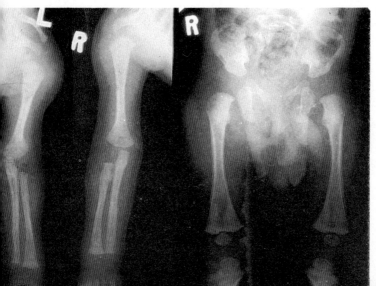426

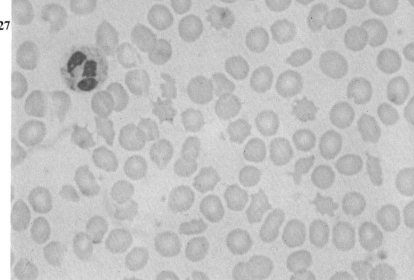

427 This patient with chronic renal failure has a haemoglobin of 9 g/dl.
  a What erythrocyte abnormality is demonstrated?
  b List five factors which may contribute to the anaemia of chronic renal failure.

428

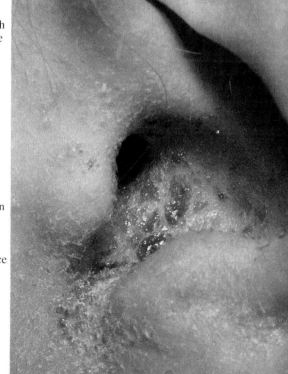

428 This North Sea saturation diver complains of pain and discharge from his left ear.
  a What is this appearance called?
  b Which organisms are likely to be responsible?
  c Is this condition preventable?

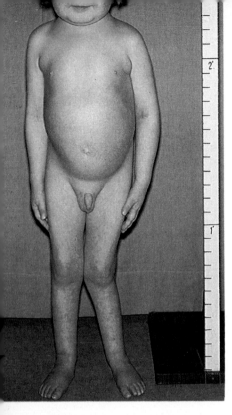

429 This four year old child
has vitamin D-resistant
rickets.
  a What physical
    abnormalities are
    visible?
  b What are the typical
    abnormalities on
    biochemical testing in
    this condition?
  c What is the likelihood
    that his younger
    brother will be
    affected?

430 This patient's Treponema
pallidum
haemagglutination
(TPHA) test is positive.
  a What name describes
    the abnormal
    appearance of her skin?
  b Suggest two possible
    diagnoses.

430

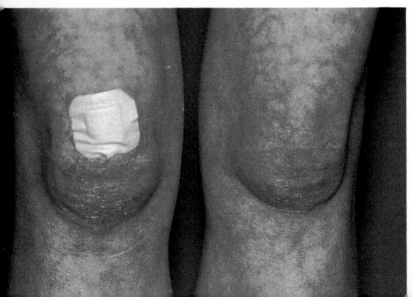

431

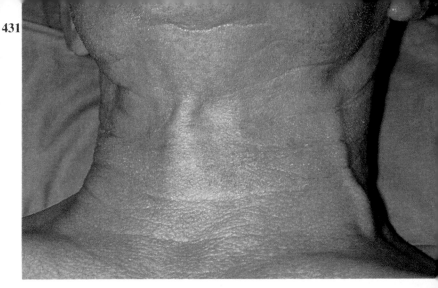

431 and 432

   a What abnormalities are seen in this patient's neck and left arm?

   b What is

      i) the diagnosis, and

      ii) the likely cause?

432

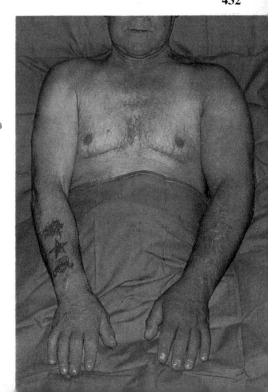

433

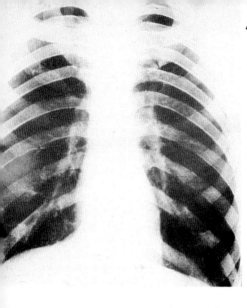

433 and 434 This man with treated hypothyroidism was admitted for investigation of weight loss and lassitude. These films were taken before and after initiation of therapy.

   a What therapy was given?

   b What is the diagnosis?

434

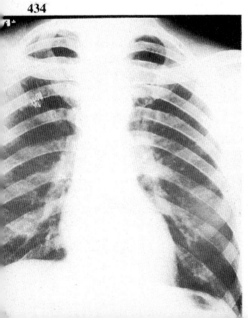

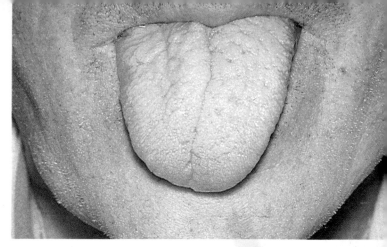

435 This man has weakness
and loss of proprioception
in his left arm and leg. He
is attempting to protrude
his tongue directly
forward.

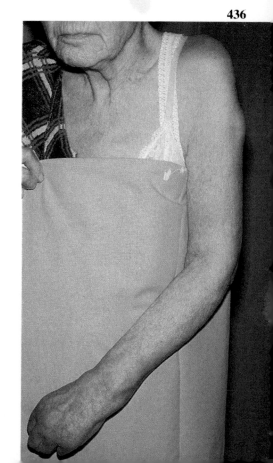

a What abnormalities of
   the tongue are present?
b Will this man's taste be
   affected?
c What is the diagnosis
   and which structures
   are involved?

436 This woman sustained a
myocardial infarction
three months ago. She has
now developed stiffness,
hyperaesthesia and
intermittent swelling of
her left arm.
a What condition has
   developed?
b What other diseases
   predispose to it?
c What therapy is
   available?

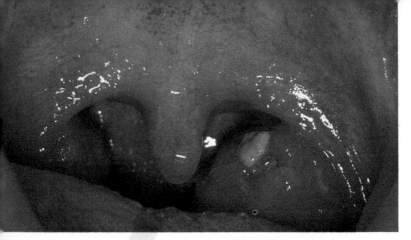

437

437 a What abnormalities are shown?
b Which infectious disease characteristically produces these appearances?

438

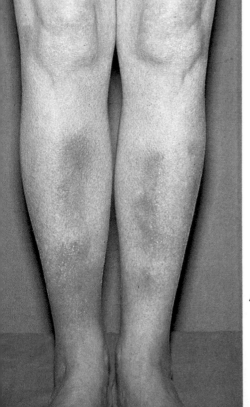

438 a What is this?
b Name two drugs commonly associated with this appearance?

439 a What is this condition?
   b What are chromosome
      studies likely to show?
   c What is the principal
      cardiovascular
      abnormality associated
      with this disorder?

440 a Other than nicotine-
      staining, what
      abnormality is shown?
   b What is likely to be the
      underlying cause?

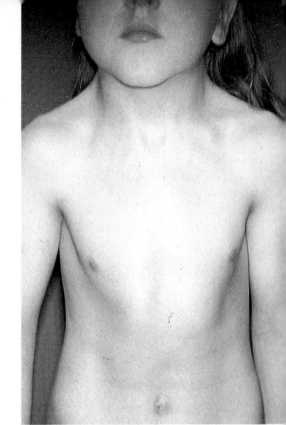

439

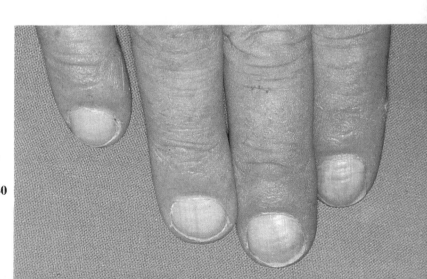

440

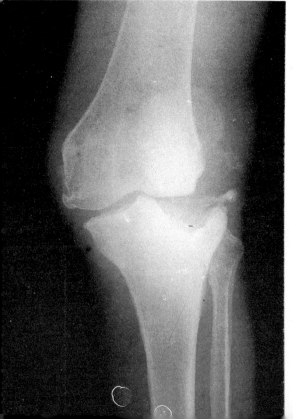

441 This lesion has been present for over five years. It is gradually increasing in size.
a What infective agent may be responsible?
b Which clinical sign may help establish the diagnosis?

442

442 What are the two commonest infective causes of this appearance?

443, 444 and 445 This patient developed a painful eruption in the areas shown.
a What is the diagnosis?
b What organism is responsible?

443

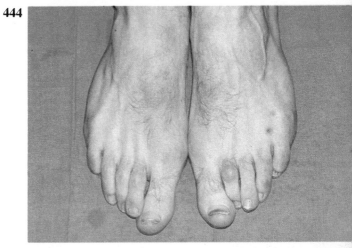

444

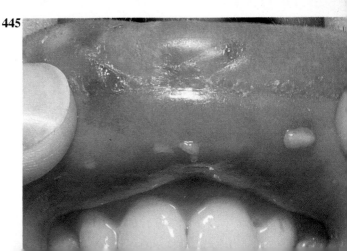

445

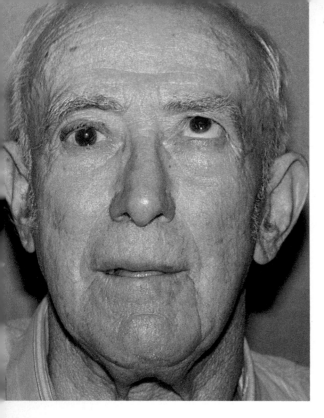

446

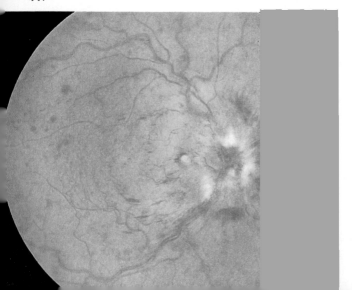

447

448

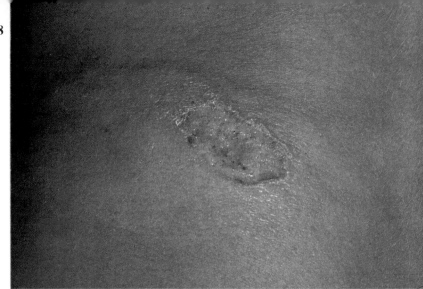

446 This man with a history of Graves' disease has been asked to look up.
  a What is the likely cause of the abnormality shown?
  b What abnormality may be detected on tonometry?

447 a What is this condition?
  b With which systemic diseases is it associated?

448 This patient originates from the Indian subcontinent. The lesion seen in his right loin has been present for four years. During that time its size has varied, but it has never completely healed. Suggest three possible infective causes.

449 This woman has erythromelalgia.
  a Of what symptoms is she likely to complain?
  b Suggest four possible underlying diagnoses.

449

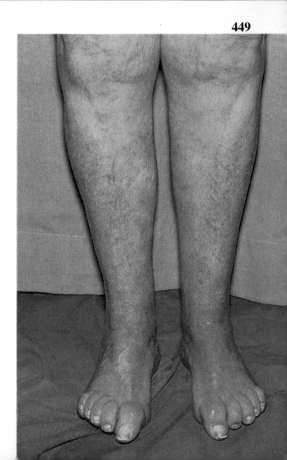

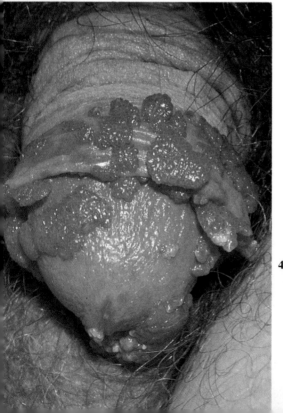

450 This man presented with a
seven day history of
headache, malaise,
anorexia, and fever. The
following day he
developed severe
diarrhoea associated with
abdominal pain.
- a What is this lesion?
- b Does it blanch on
pressure?
- c What other clinical
abdominal findings
may be detected?

451

451 These are condylomata
acuminata.
- a Is dark ground
microscopy of help in
establishing the
diagnosis?
- b What forms of therapy
are available?

452 This man has a three year history of cardiac failure and persistent heavy proteinuria (4g/24 hours). He has recently developed left renal angle pain, haematuria, followed by pleuritic chest pain and haemoptysis.

a What is the likely cause of his loin pain?

b How is this thought to occur?

c What is the underlying diagnosis?

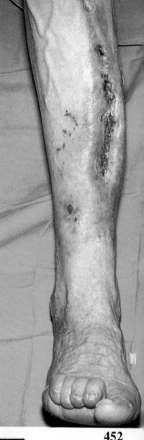

452

453 Name six infections which may cause this appearance.

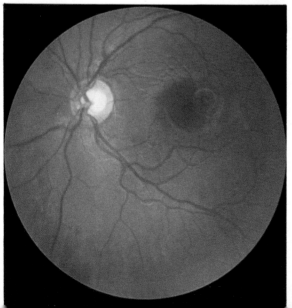

453

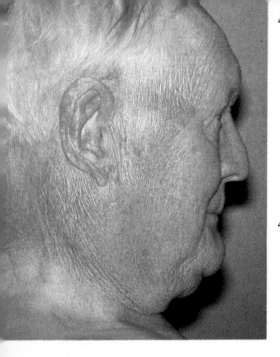

455

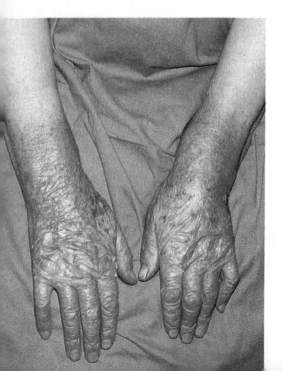

454 and 455 This patient complains of recurrent facial flushing and wheezing, and of frequent diarrhoea with colicky abdominal pain. For the past two months he has been aware of a rash affecting his hands and face as shown. Abdominal examination reveals hepatomegaly. There is an ejection systolic murmur, loudest in the second left interspace.

a What deficiency state may have given rise to the patient's rash?

b What is the underlying diagnosis?

c How is this diagnosis established biochemically?

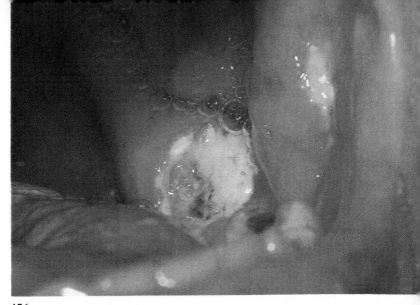

456

456 This patient suffers from recurrent migratory superficial thrombophlebitis usually affecting the calf veins.
  a What abnormality is seen in the buccal mucosa?
  b Which diagnosis does this suggest?
  c List three other typical manifestations of thrombophlebitis in this condition.

457

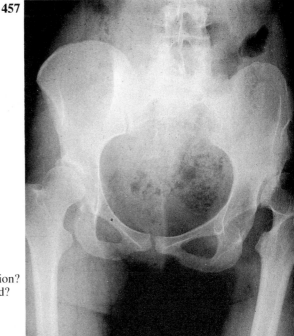

457 a What is this condition?
   b Can it be prevented?

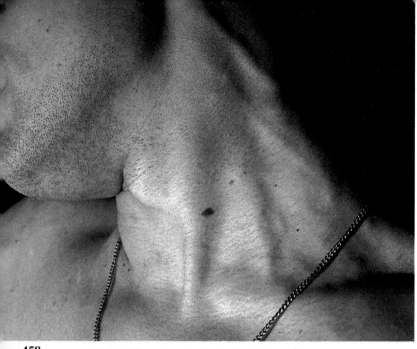

458

458 a What abnormality is shown?
  b List five conditions which can give rise to this appearance.

459 This woman has a history of erythema nodosum. She now presents with
  an anterior uveitis.
  a What complication has developed?
  b Which systemic diseases may present with these features?

459

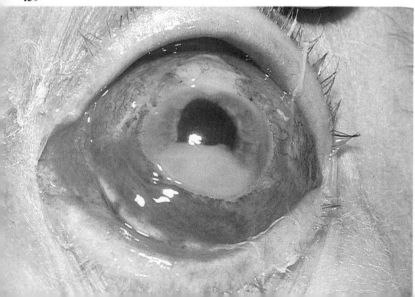

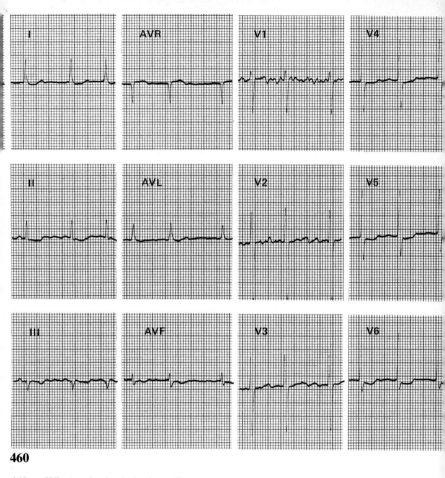

460

460 a What arrhythmia is shown?
  b List six predisposing factors.

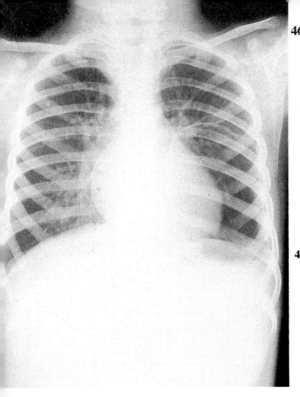

461 This is the chest x-ray of an asymptomatic man.
  a What abnormality is present in this chest x-ray and what is the likely diagnosis?
  b What is the aetiology of this condition?
  c Which clinical sign is usually detectable?

462 This patient has recurrent episodes of acholuric jaundice. Alkaline phosphatase, aspartate aminotransferase and gamma glutamyl transferase activities are normal. Haemoglobin is 12 g/dl.
  a What is the likely diagnosis?
  b What feature of liver histology is typical of this condition?
  c Suggest two alternative diagnoses.

462

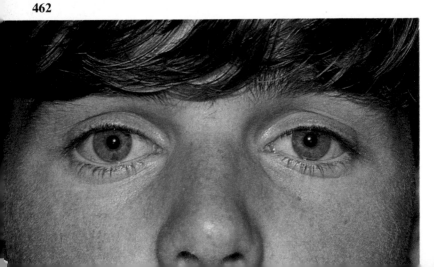

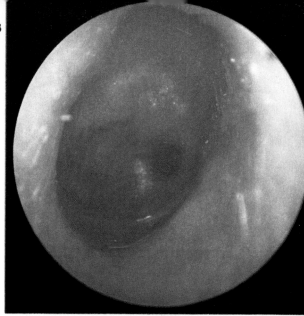

463 a What is the diagnosis?
b Which organisms are
usually responsible?

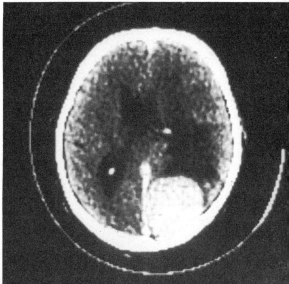

464 This fifty-nine year old
woman complained of
poor vision in her left eye
and was noted to have a
left homonymous
hemianopia. The CT scan
has been performed after
administration of
contrast.
a Will her hemianopia
spare the macula?
b What is the most likely
nature of the lesion
seen in the CT scan?

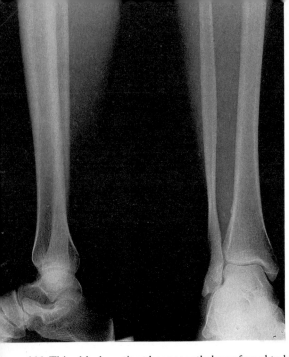

465 This forty-five year old East African patient presents with a focal seizure which progressed to a grand mal convulsion. There is no previous history of seizures. Skull x-ray is normal.

  a What abnormality is seen in this x-ray?

  b What should be considered as a possible cause of the seizure?

  c Which antimicrobial agent may be indicated?

466 This elderly patient has recently been found to be diabetic, requiring insulin therapy. Despite reasonable control of blood glucose she has continued to lose weight. She complains of recurrent episodes of pain and tenderness in the calves, and more recently in the left arm. The affected area is shown.

  a What is the cause of her leg and arm symptoms?

  b What is a probable cause of her weight loss?

466

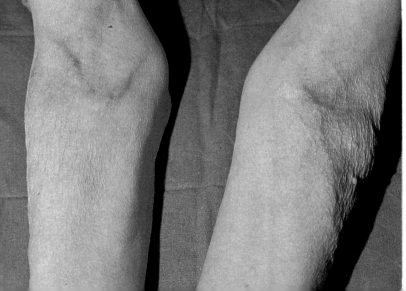

467

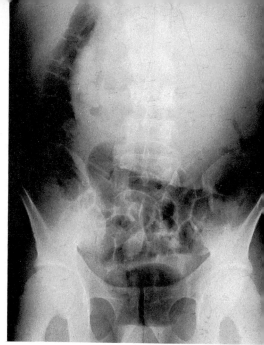

467 a What principal
abnormality is seen on
this abdominal x-ray?
b List five causes of this
appearance.

468 a What name is given to the lesions seen on this asymptomatic
middle-aged patient's back?
b What is their significance?

468

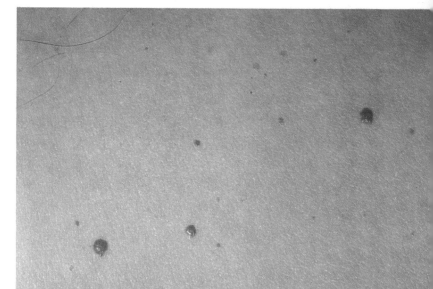

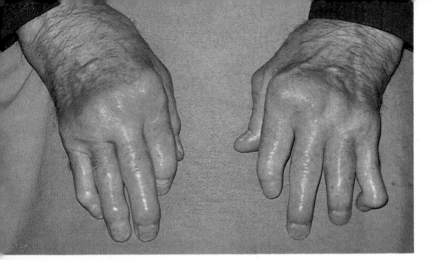

469

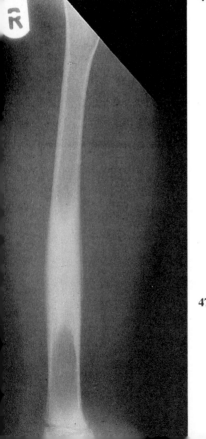

470

469 a With which skin disease is this arthropathy associated?
b What other forms of arthropathy may occur in this condition?
c Are chloroquine or hydroxychloroquine useful drugs in this condition?

470 This patient has sickle cell anaemia.
a What complication has developed?
b Which agent is typically responsible for this complication?

471
This woman's visual
acuity has been
deteriorating steadily.
She is otherwise well. She
has neither clinical nor
biochemical evidence of
diabetes mellitus.
a What is the diagnosis?
b What treatment may be
   useful?
c What abnormality of
   her visual fields would
   be detected on
   confrontation testing?

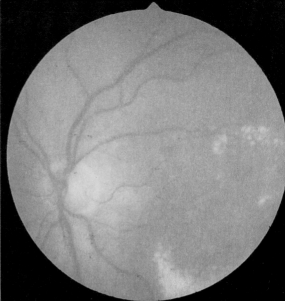

472 This painful lesion developed on the hand after the patient had been
helping with lambing.
a What is the diagnosis?
b What complications may occur?

472

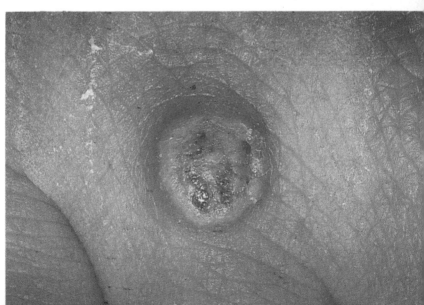

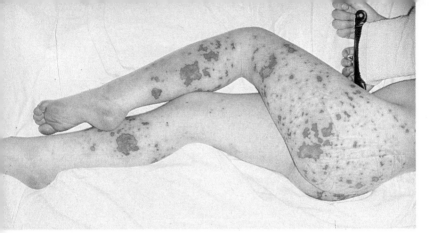

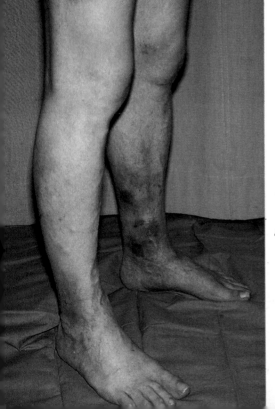

473 This girl complained of malaise and severe headache, before becoming increasingly drowsy and unresponsive. On admission she was moribund.
 a What is the likely diagnosis?
 b What drug therapy is indicated?
 c What would her plasma cortisol level be?

474 This man has had recurrent deep venous thromboses. His father and one brother have had similar problems.
 a What sequelae have developed?
 b Name two hereditary conditions which may produce this picture.

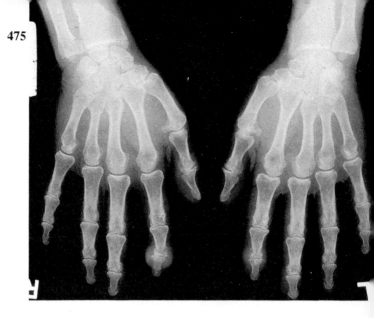

475

475 and 476
  a What condition is this?
  b What is the main
     hazard of commencing
     this man on a xanthine
     oxidase inhibitor?
  c What is the significance
     of Autumn crocuses in
     this disease?

476

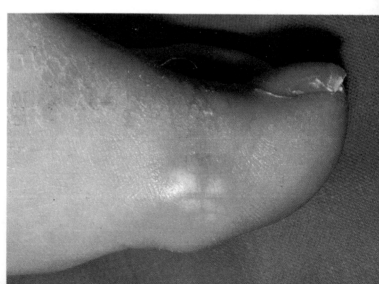

477 This patient complains of undue itching and weal formation after skin scratching.
  a What phenomenon is shown?
  b What is the main mediator of this reaction?

477

478

478 a This patient noted these painless lesions on his penis. What is the diagnosis?
  b By what means is this best established?

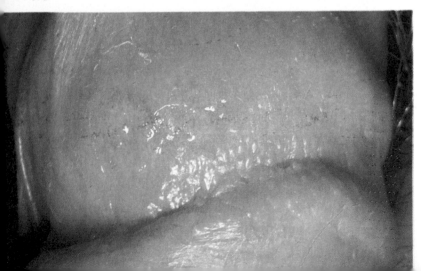

479 a What abnormalities are
seen here?
b What is the diagnosis?

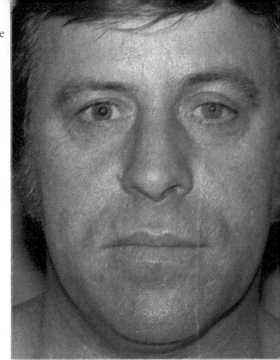

479

480 a Describe the
abnormalities present
in this optic fundus.
b What is the likely
underlying disorder?

480

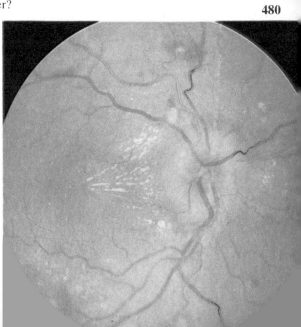

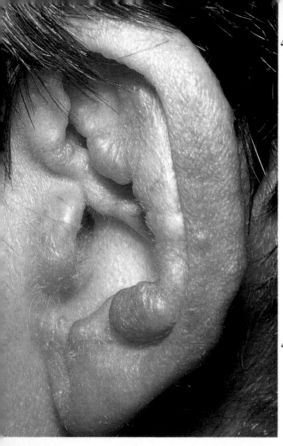

481 and 482 This patient complains of joint pains suggestive of acute gout. His serum uric acid, however, is persistently normal and uric acid crystals are not present in the synovial fluid of an inflamed joint.
What is the unusual cause of his symptoms?

482

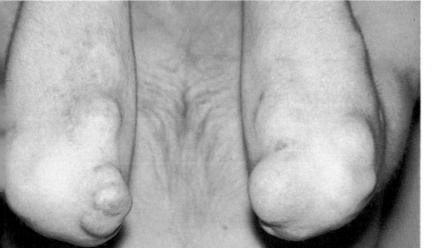

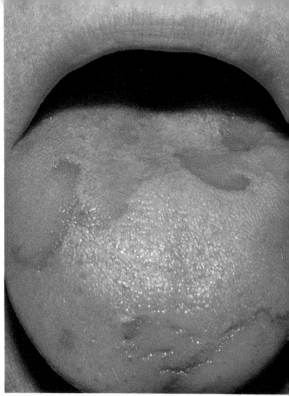

483 What serological
abnormalities are
suggested by this
appearance, and why?

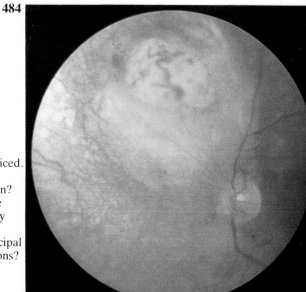

484 This patient is jaundiced.
  a What fundal
    abnormality is seen?
  b Which layer of the
    eyeball is primarily
    affected?
  c What are the principal
    ocular complications?

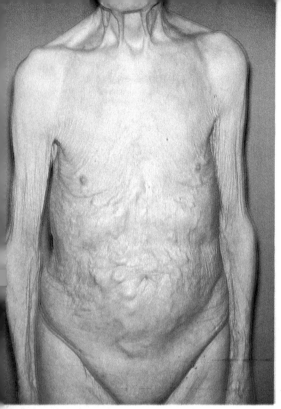

485 a What principal
abnormality is seen on
this elderly male
patient's abdomen?
b What is the likely
cause?

486 a What abnormality is
seen in this neonate's
hand?
b Which congenital
disorder is most usually
associated with this
abnormality?
c Which other abnormal
appearance of the hand
is commonly seen in
this disorder?

486

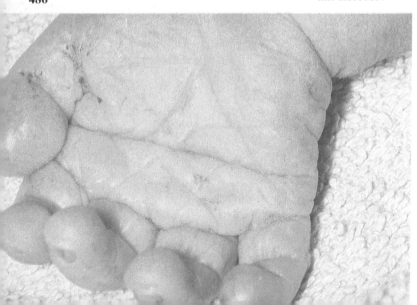

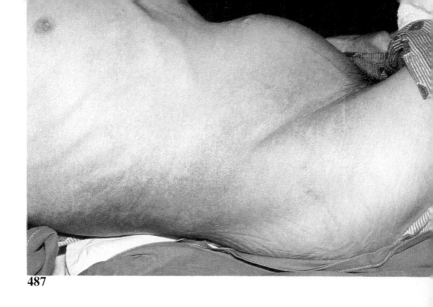

487

488

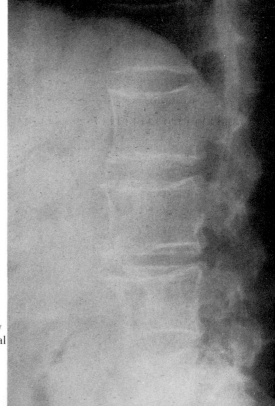

487 and 488
- a What principal abnormality is seen on this patient's trunk?
- b What radiological abnormality is visible?
- c What is the most likely underlying pathological condition?

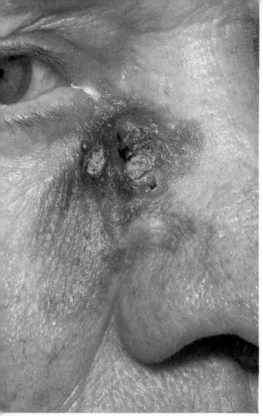

489 The lesion seen on this
elderly patient's face has
recently changed in
appearance. Spontaneous
bleeding has occurred.
 a What name is given to
  the original lesion?
 b What complication has
  developed?

489

490 This asymptomatic lesion
has been present for
several months. There are
no other skin or mucosal
abnormalities.
What are the two
principal differential
diagnoses?

490

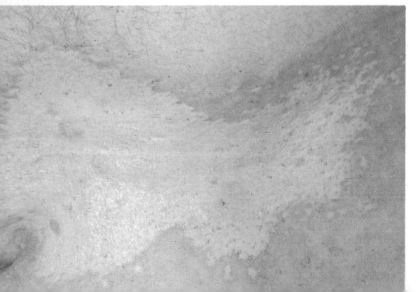

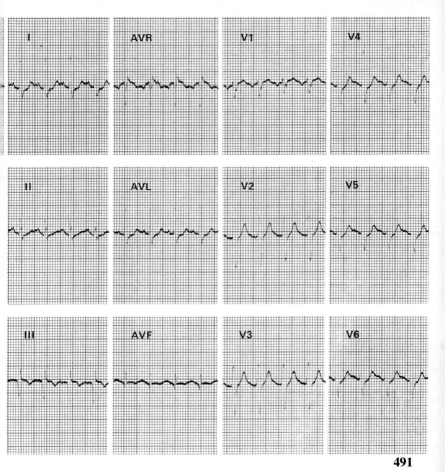

491

491 This fifty-six year old man was admitted with a suspected right lower lobe pneumonia. ECG on admission was normal and the trace shown was recorded fifteen hours later.
a What significant changes have developed?
b What is the likely diagnosis?
c What immediate treatment is indicated?

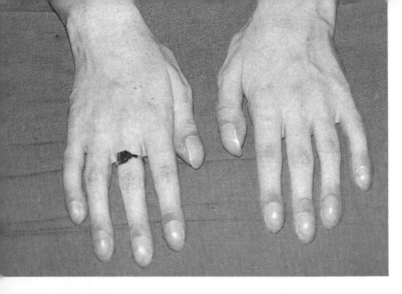

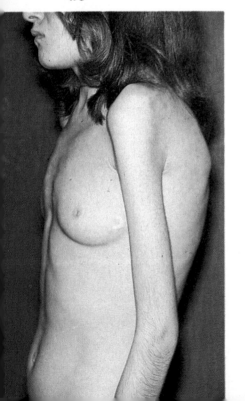

493

492 and 493 This girl has a history of recurrent chest infection, recurrent acute abdominal pain and steatorrhoea. Diabetes mellitus has recently been diagnosed.

a What abnormalities are seen of
  i)   the chest?
  ii) the hands?
b What is the likely diagnosis?
c What treatment is indicated for the cause of her steatorrhoea?

494

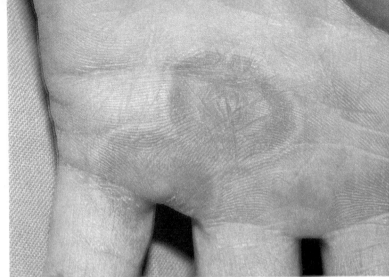

494 This twenty-eight year old patient presented with a dry cough of ten days duration. Her chest was clear to auscultation and no antibiotic was prescribed. The cough persisted and she developed a widespread rash. For the past day she has been passing increasingly dark urine which produces a positive result for blood on stick testing, but which contains no red cells.
   a Describe the morphology of the lesion shown.
   b What rash has she developed?
   c What is the cause of her urinary abnormality?
   d What is the underlying diagnosis?
   e What serological
      tests would support
      this diagnosis?

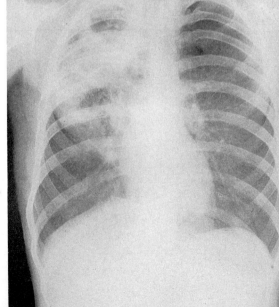

495 This patient is diabetic.
   a What abnormality is
      seen in the chest x-ray?
   b What are the two most
      likely causes in this
      patient?
   c Suggest three other
      general causes of such
      appearances.

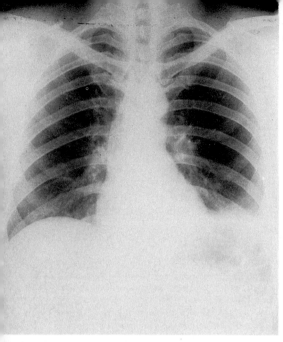

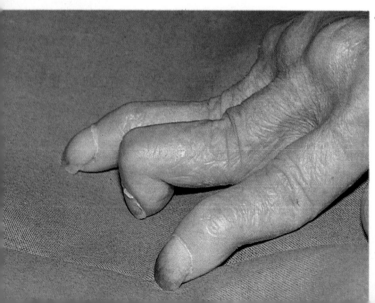

496 and 497
  a What is the association between these conditions?
  b What are the biochemical and microscopic characteristics of the principal extra-articular abnormality seen on this radiograph?
  c What is this joint deformity called and how does it occur?

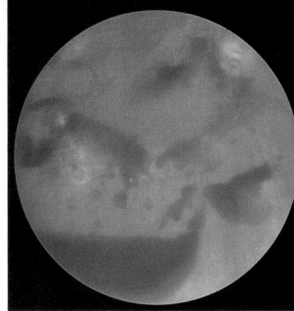

498 This insulin dependent diabetic complained of sudden loss of vision in his left eye.
    a What is this appearance?
    b To what is it usually secondary?
    c What complications may ensue?

499 a What is this lesion?
    b What is the most important histological feature from the point of view of prognosis?

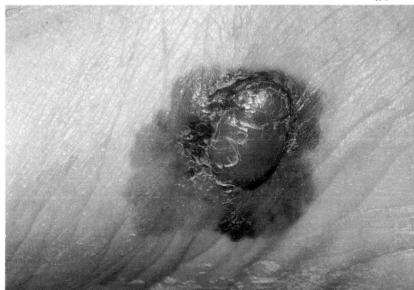

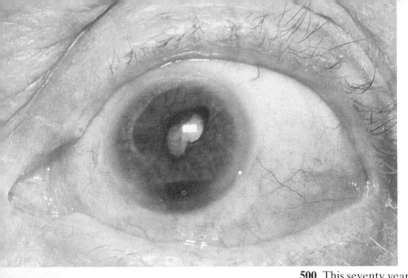

500 This seventy year old
patient whose visual
acuity in this eye has been
poor for several years,
now complains of sudden
blindness in the eye.
  a List five abnormalities
    seen in the eye.
  b What is the likely cause
    of the sudden visual
    deterioration?

501

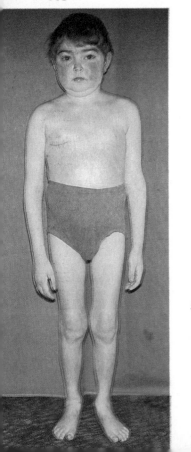

501 a Describe the
abnormalities seen in
this twelve year old
boy.
  b What is the likely
    diagnosis?
  c List three possible
    causes.

502

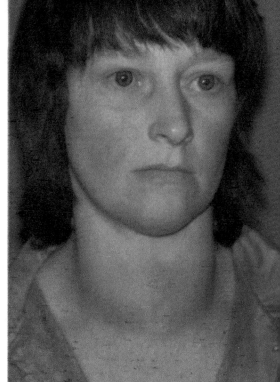

502 a What physical
abnormality does this
young woman show?
b What is the likely
diagnosis?
c Suggest four
investigations that you
might carry out to
establish a diagnosis.

503

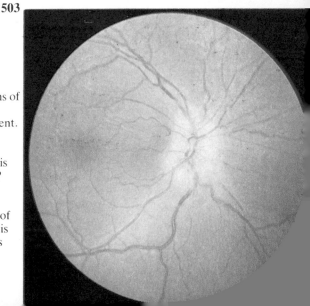

503 This patient complains of
pain behind the eye,
worse on eye movement.
He has no other
complaints.
a What abnormality is
seen in the fundus?
b What is the likely
diagnosis?
c What abnormality of
pupillary response is
associated with this
condition?

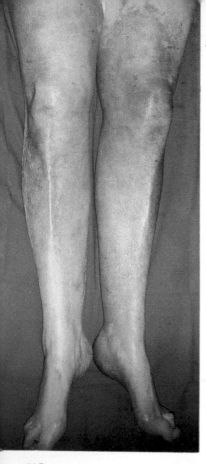

504

504 This patient recently suffered a myocardial infarction, complicated by fast atrial fibrillation resistant to digitalisation. Direct current cardioversion was successfully carried out. Shortly afterwards she complained of pain and coldness of the legs.
a What is the cause of her symptoms?
b What urgent treatment is necessary?

505

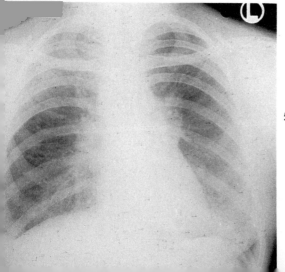

505 a What name is given to the abnormality seen in the lung fields?
b Two other abnormalities are visible on the chest x-ray. List these and suggest a diagnosis which links all three.

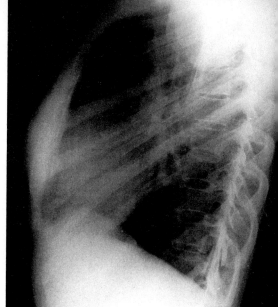

506 a What abnormality is seen in this lateral chest x-ray?
b Give three possible causes of such lesions in this area.

507 This twenty-five year old male is deeply unconscious, making no response to painful stimuli. There are no lateralising CNS signs but his pupils are pinpoint, and his respirations shallow.
a What abnormality is seen on the skin of his forearm?
b What single therapeutic manoeuvre may be life saving here?

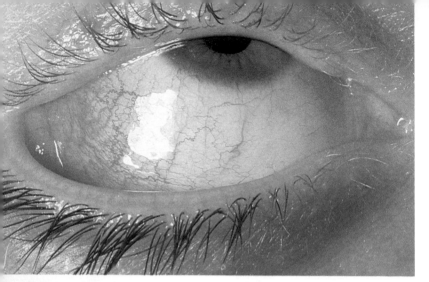

508

508 This patient complains of constant dull ache in the eye. He has been asked to look up.
  a What is the diagnosis?
  b With which non-ocular disorders may this be associated?

509

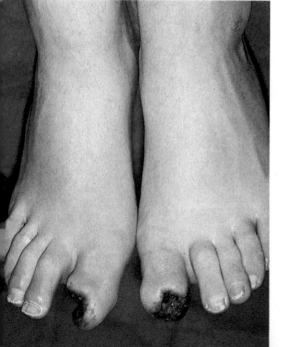

509 This patient has been an insulin-dependent diabetic for twenty years.
  a What principal abnormality is seen in the feet?
  b What is the likely precipitant?

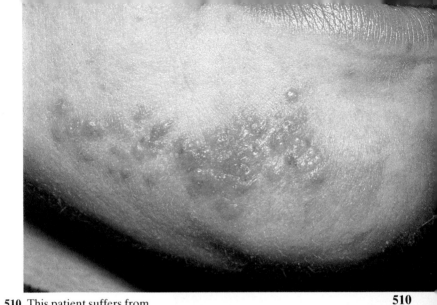

510 This patient suffers from recurrent cold sores of the chin.

  a What complication of these has occurred?

  b What are the usual causative agents of the complicating condition?

511 The abnormality seen in this patient's scalp is known as pseudopelade. Which two systemic disorders may predispose to this condition?

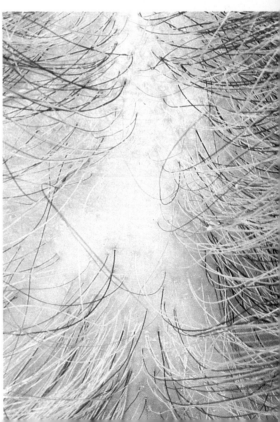

510

511

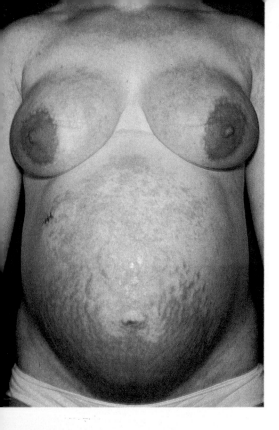

512 This patient's bullous rash
has been present
throughout most of her
pregnancy.
a What is the likely
diagnosis?
b What is the causative
agent?
c Is the rash likely to
recur in successive
pregnancies?

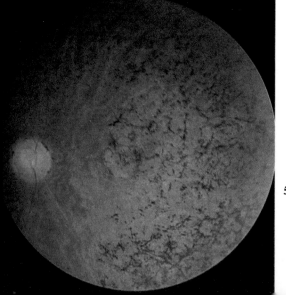

513 a What is this condition?
b Of what is the patient
likely to complain?

514 This patient complains of
tinnitus in the right ear.
The right corneal reflex is
absent. He has been
asked to close his eyes.
a What is the most likely
diagnosis?
b Give two reasons why
Bell's palsy is unlikely.

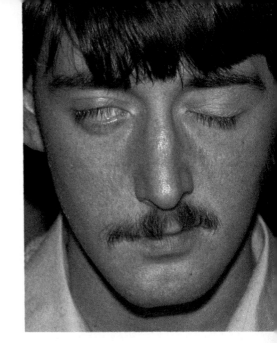

514

515 This patient has iron
deficiency anaemia.
a What unusual diagnosis
is suggested by the
appearance of her lips?
b What is the
characteristic
association in this
condition?
c Her husband is
unaffected. What is the
likelihood that her son
will have this disorder?

515

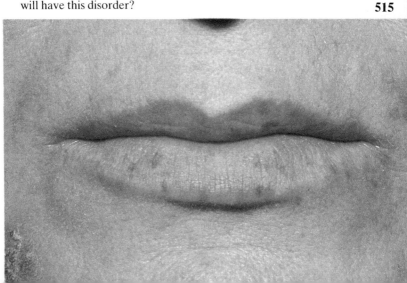

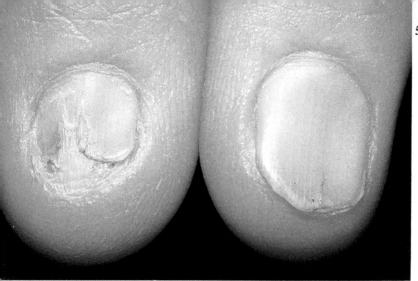

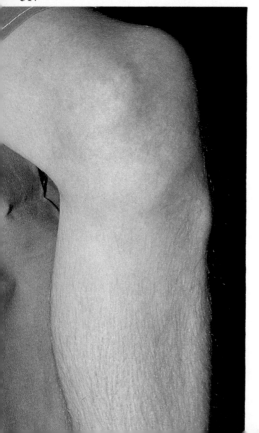

516 and 517 This patient's
   urinalysis is abnormal.
   a What principal
     abnormality is seen in
     i)   the finger nails?
     ii) the knee?
   b What is the diagnosis?
   c What abnormality of
     the urine is likely?

518

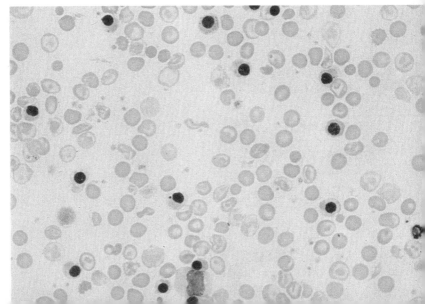

518 This child was playing alone happily at home when she suddenly became breathless and cyanosed. There is no significant previous medical history.
  a What two principal abnormalities are seen in the chest x-ray?
  b What is the likely diagnosis?

519 This Greek-Cypriot girl requires regular blood transfusion.
  a What abnormalities are present on this blood film?
  b What is the diagnosis?
  c What therapy should she receive in addition to her blood transfusion?

519

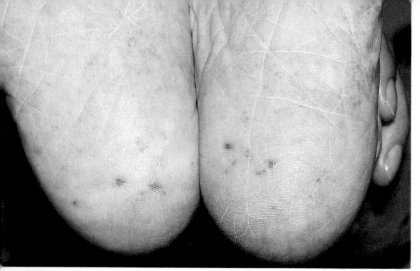

520

521

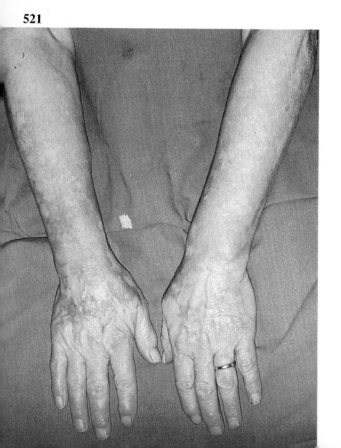

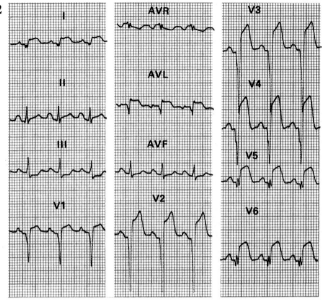

520 This patient complains of weight loss and malaise. She has a low grade fever and a mild normochromic normocytic anaemia. An early diastolic murmur is present at the left sternal border.

    a What name is given to the asymptomatic abnormality seen on her soles?

    b What is the likely diagnosis?

521 This patient is concerned about the cosmetic appearance of her skin.

    a What is this condition?

    b What forms of therapy are available?

522 a What is the diagnosis?

    b What are the three major indications for anticoagulant therapy in this condition?

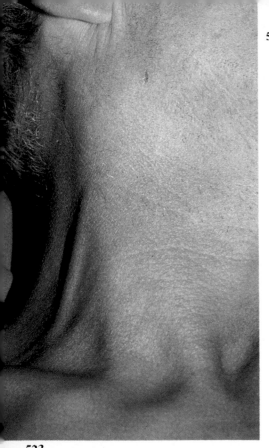

523 a What is shown here?
    b What implication can
      be drawn about mean
      right atrial pressure?

524 a What principal features
    does the illustration
    demonstrate?
    b What is the diagnosis?
    c Which joints in the
      hand are typically
      affected?

523

524

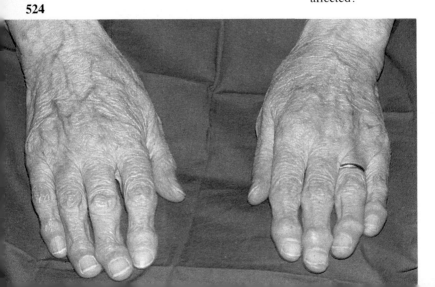

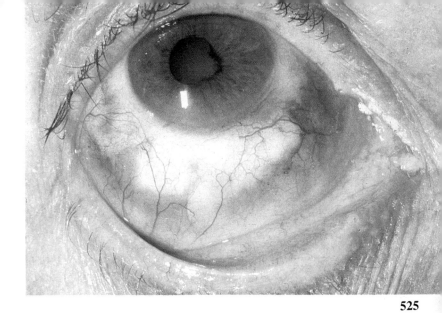

525

525 This patient has an
inflammatory joint
disorder.

   a In addition to the
irregular pupil, what
abnormality is shown
here?

   b With which joint
disease is this typically
associated?

526

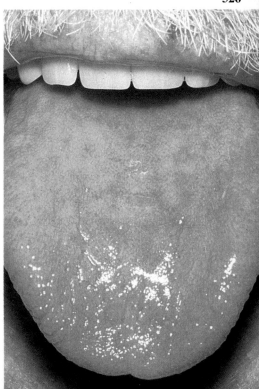

526 This patient complains of
unsteadiness and of pins
and needles in his feet.
He has a history of gastric
surgery.
What might be the
findings in his peripheral
blood film?

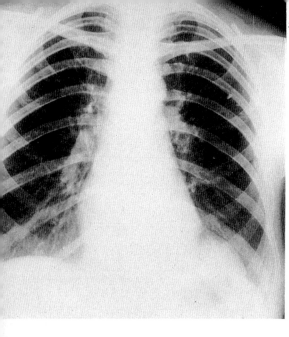

527 a What is the most likely
cause of this
appearance?
b Name two conditions
which may produce a
similar appearance.

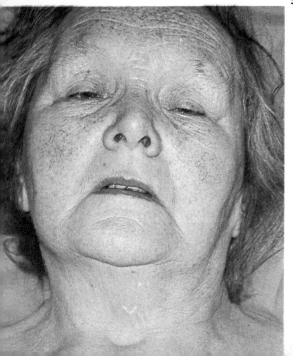

528 This patient was found at
home, collapsed and
hypothermic. Her rectal
temperature is 32°C and
blood pressure 90/60. She
is drowsy but rousable,
although disorientated
when wakened. There are
no localising neurological
signs, but her deep
tendon reflexes are
generally depressed. She
is on no regular
medication.
a What endocrine
diagnosis is suggested
by her facial
appearance?
b List five biochemical
features of this disorder
which may be
contributing to her
clinical state.

529 This patient complains of increasing pain in this finger for three days.
  a What is this condition?
  b What is the usual causative agent?
  c What would be the most appropriate therapy?

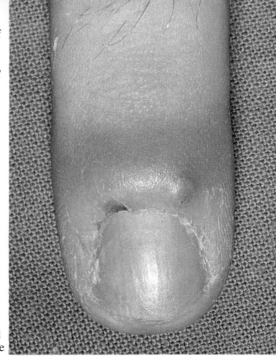

529

530 a What abnormality is present in this cerebral CT scan and what is the most likely diagnosis?
  b What signs are likely to be present?
  c What abnormality of conjugate eye movements may be present?

530

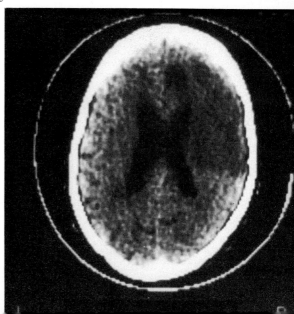

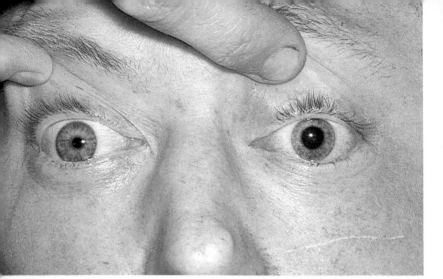

531

532

531 This man complained of
left retro-orbital pain and
diplopia. He then
developed more severe
headache with loss of
consciousness.
  a What is the probable
    diagnosis?
  b Why is this unlikely to
    be a Horner's
    syndrome?
  c How is the diagnosis
    best confirmed?

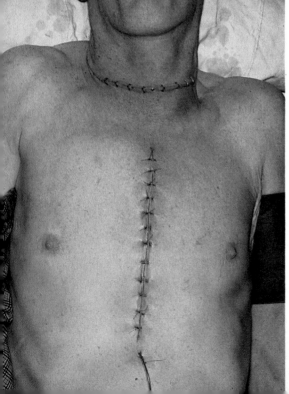

532 This fifty year old man
presented with increasing
weakness, intermittent
diplopia and swallowing
difficulty.
  a What operation has
    been performed? For
    what indication?
  b What abnormalities
    may the involved organ
    show?
  c Should he develop a
    post-operative
    infection, which drugs
    are best avoided?

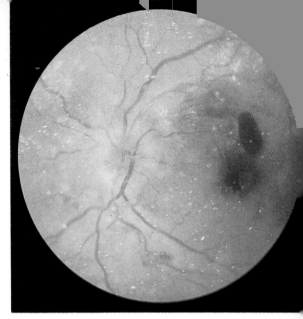

533 This patient has chronic renal failure.
a What abnormalities are present?
b What is the most likely cause of the fundal abnormalities?

534 This forty-year old woman has a history of painful fingers since her teens. Her fingers blanch particularly on exposure to cold, then become painful and red. Her mother has a similar problem.
a What is this condition?
b What is the likelihood of her developing trophic changes in her digits?
c Which drugs should she avoid?

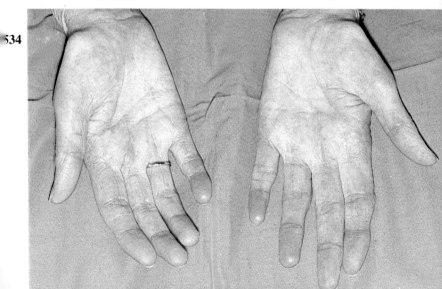

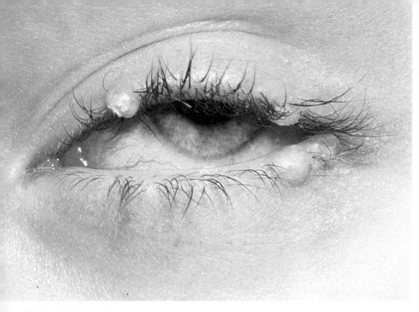

535 a What is this infective lesion?
   b Is the patient's vision at risk?

536 a Which underlying nutritional disorder is suggested by the abnormal appearance of this child's ankles?
   b List four other clinical features of this disorder.

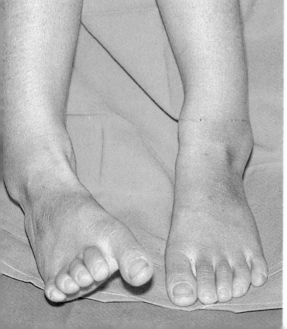

536

537

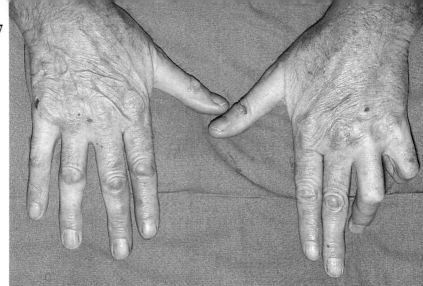

537 This elderly patient complains of a recent blistering eruption on his hands particularly during the summer months. He has been asked to place his hands flat.
  a What is the probable cause of the deformity of the left hand?
  b What is the likely cause of his rash?
  c How is this skin condition inherited?
  d What are the mainstays of treatment of the skin disorder?

538

538 A recent routine chest x-ray revealed a regular opacity in this patient's right lower lobe. On questioning he remembered coughing up an unusual quantity of thin salty fluid some months ago, but has otherwise been symptom free. Following computerised tomography he proceeded to surgery: the appearances at thoracotomy are shown.
  a What is the most likely cause of this lesion?
  b By what means is this condition usually contracted?
  c What is the major hazard of surgery of this condition?

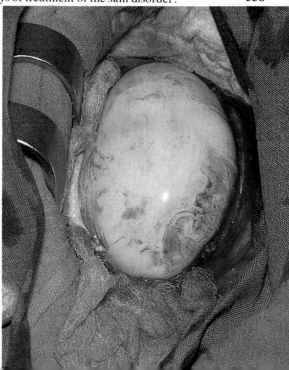

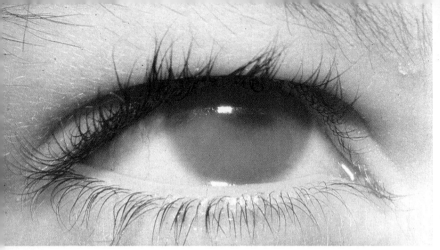

539

540

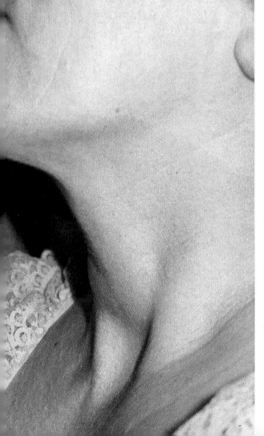

539 This child suffers from an inherited disorder of metabolism.
  a What ocular abnormality is seen?
  b What diagnosis does this suggest?
  c Which substances are found in excessive quantities in the urine of these patients?

540 This patient received x-ray treatment as a teenager to a birthmark on her neck. She complains of recent onset of pain in and development of a hard lump in the neck.
  a What diagnosis should be suspected?
  b What would you expect to see on isotope scan?

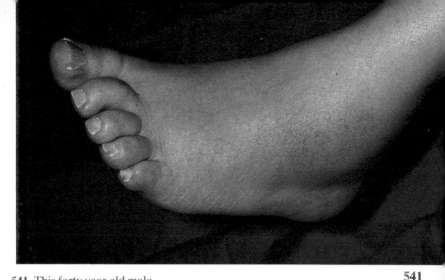

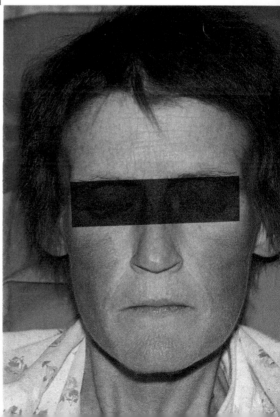

541 This forty year old male presents with an acutely painful ankle. He has no other joint symptoms but feels generally unwell and is pyrexial. Four weeks ago a combination of atenolol and chlorthalidone was prescribed because of recently diagnosed essential hypertension.

a What is the most likely diagnosis?

b What is the principal differential diagnosis?

c What investigation is mandatory?

542 a With which form of valvular heart disease is this facial appearance typically associated?

b What changes in auscultatory findings accompany increasing severity of this lesion?

c Which single invasive measurement best defines the severity of the lesion?

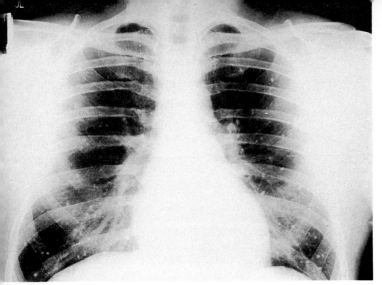

543

544

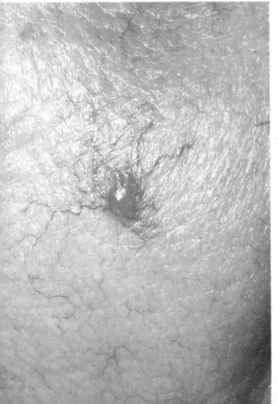

543 This chest x-ray was taken as part of this patient's insurance medical examination. He has no cardiorespiratory symptoms.
  a What abnormality is seen in the lung fields?
  b Give three infective causes of these appearances.

544 a What is this?
  b With which three principal conditions are such lesions associated?

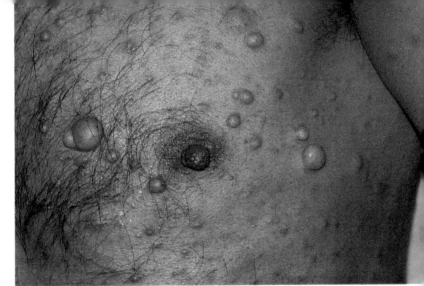

545 This patient is hypertensive.
  a What condition is shown here?
  b Which underlying disorder should be considered?
  c What is the usual mode of inheritance of the condition shown?

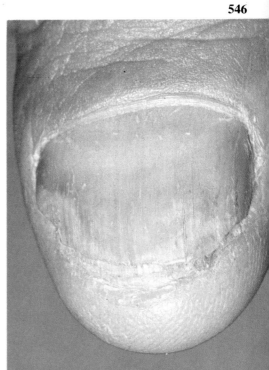

546 a Name this sign.
  b List five causes.

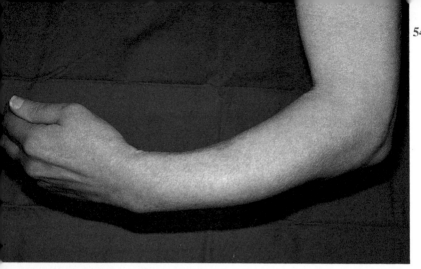

547 The abnormal appearance of this thirty-five year old woman's arm has been present for several months.
What is the most likely cause of this abnormality?

548 This appearance has been present since birth.
  a What is this condition?
  b What effect may this have on vision?

548

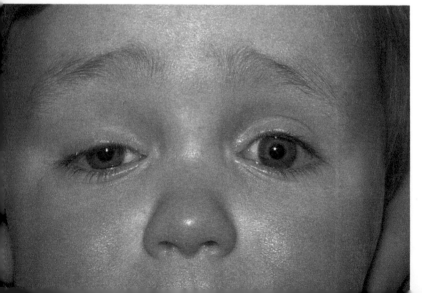

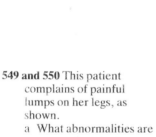

549 and 550 This patient complains of painful lumps on her legs, as shown.

a What abnormalities are seen on her chest x-ray?

b What is the likely diagnosis?

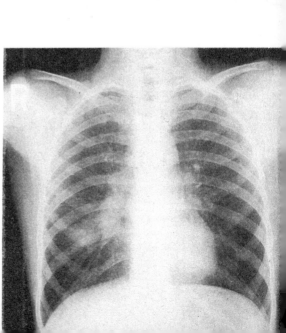

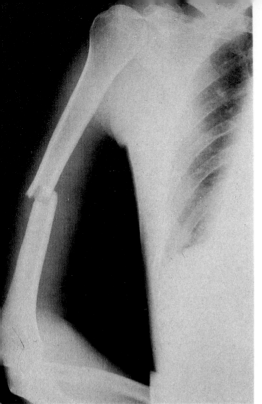

551

a What abnormality is seen in this x-ray?

b Which nerve is most likely to be damaged?

c What neurological abnormalities would this produce?

553 The lesion, on this patient's trunk, has been gradually spreading outwards for several months.

a What is this condition?

b What is its cause?

c What is the most appropriate oral therapy?

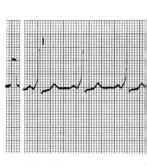

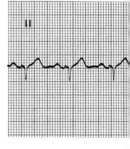

552 This is the ECG of a twenty-nine year old man referred for investigation of fits.

a What abnormalities are present?

b What is the diagnosis?

c How may this explain his fits?

552

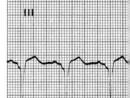

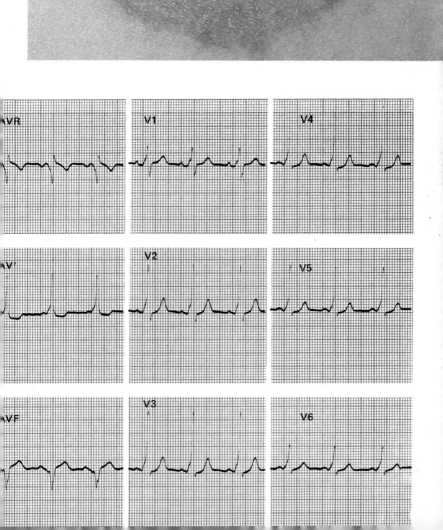

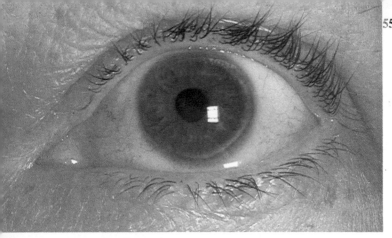

554 a What abnormality is shown?
    b With which specific biochemical abnormality is it associated?
    c With which other parameter is it positively associated?

555 This thirty year old woman presented with morning headaches of
increasing severity over the preceding six weeks. Examination was
normal apart from this fundal appearance in both eyes. CT scan was
normal. Lumbar puncture revealed acellular, sterile cerebrospinal fluid
with normal protein content and raised pressure.
    a What is the likely diagnosis?
    b What drugs may cause this condition?

555

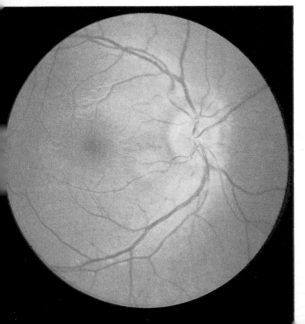

556 This patient is a hairdresser.
What is the lesion shown?

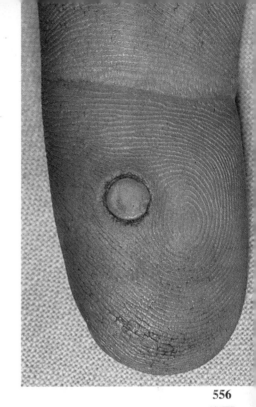

556

557 This elderly steroid-dependent asthmatic was admitted to a general medical ward. A provisional diagnosis of acute myocardial infarction had been made before admission. On examination he was pale, sweaty and hypotensive. Heart rate was 130/min. A working diagnosis of cardiogenic shock was made and dopamine infusion commenced.
a What abnormality is seen in the chest x-ray?
b What is the likely cause of his acute illness?

557

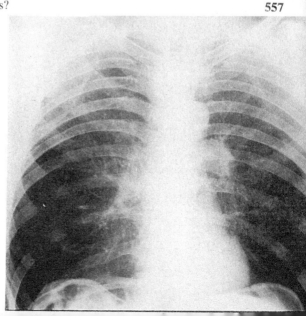

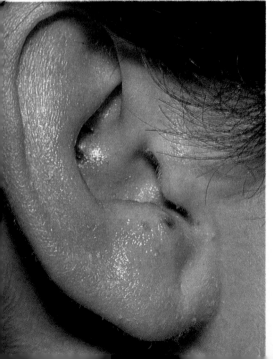

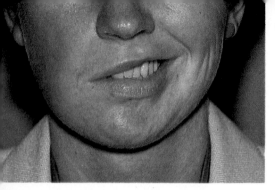

558

558 and 559 This woman complained of pain in her ear a day before this appearance developed.

   a What is the diagnosis?

   b Which other cranial nerves may be involved in this condition?

   c What degree of recovery may she expect to obtain?

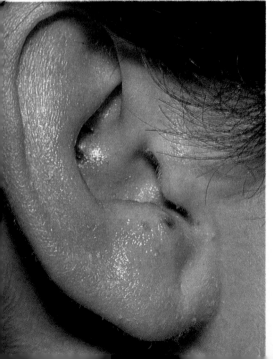

559

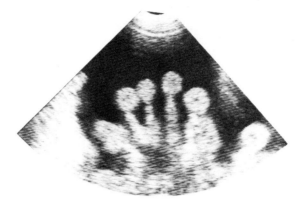

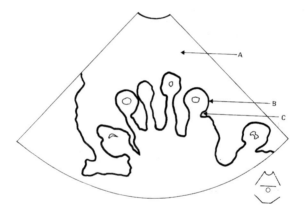

560 A known alcoholic presents with rapidly increasing abdominal
distension and anorexia.
The transverse ultrasonic abdominal scan demonstrates normal
anatomical features which have been enhanced by the presence of an
abnormality.
a Name the structures labelled 'A', 'B' and 'C'.
b Explain why the normal anatomy is so well seen in this case.

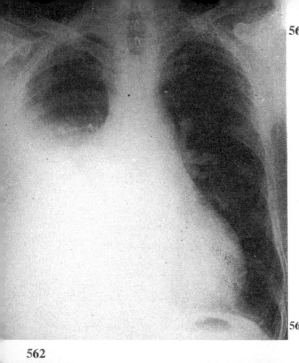

562

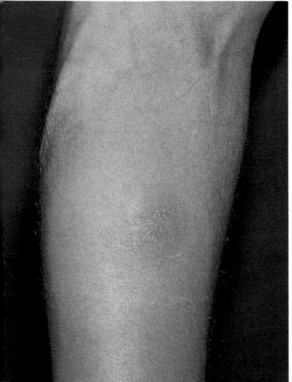

561 and 562 This eighteen year old mentally defective boy living in a children's home was noted to become increasingly breathless.
a What is the diagnosis?
b What is the likelihood of culturing the causative organism?

563

This patient complains of progressive hearing loss.

a What underlying cause is suggested by his facial appearance?

b What response would you expect to Rinne test?

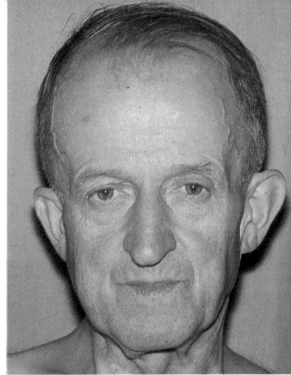

563

564 This female patient complains of persistent swelling of her legs despite several weeks of diuretic therapy. She also noticed that her nails have become discoloured and appear to have stopped growing.

a What nail abnormality is present?

b What cause for her leg swelling does this suggest?

564

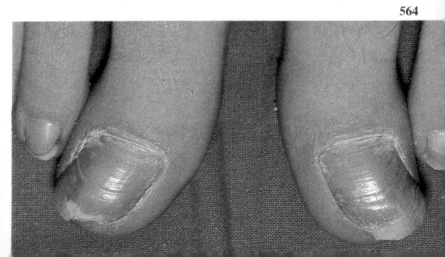

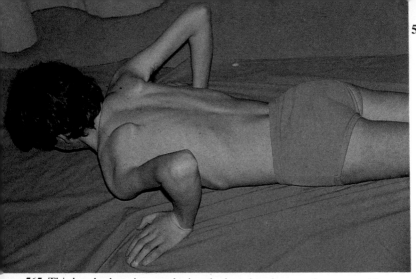

565 This boy had to give up playing the bagpipes because he was unable to keep the bag inflated. He is attempting a press-up.
a What is this condition?
b How is it acquired?
c Will he develop pelvic girdle weakness?

566 This elderly patient's elbow became acutely painful and swollen. X-ray of the elbow showed no abnormality other than soft tissue swelling. Aspiration of synovial fluid from the elbow led to a diagnosis.
a What abnormality is seen in the knees?
b What is the cause of his elbow symptoms?
c What was found in the synovial fluid?

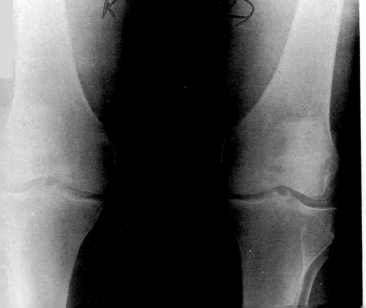

566

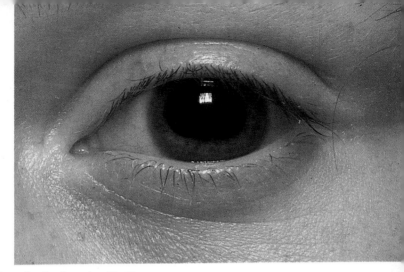

567 Atropine has been instilled into this girl's eye.
  a What abnormality is shown?
  b What is the underlying diagnosis?
  c Her ocular disease followed a severe episode of diarrhoea. What
     diagnoses should be considered?

568 This patient suffers from a chronic scaling eruption. The unusual
appearance of the abdominal scar was noticed two weeks after
operation.
  a What name is given to this phenomenon?
  b In which other circumstances may similar changes occur?
  c List four skin disorders in which this phenomenon occurs.   **568**

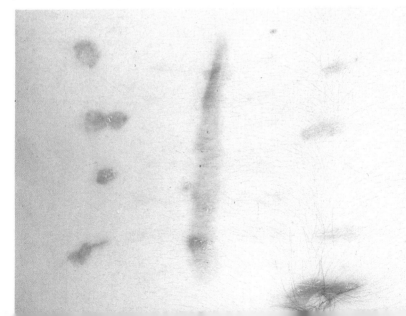

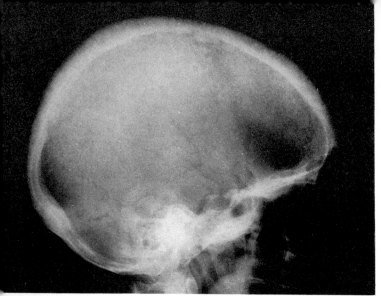

569

570

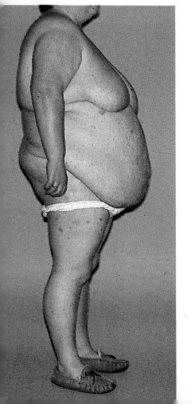

569 This patient presented with acute severe epigastric pain radiating through to the back.
a What abnormality is seen in the skull x-ray?
b What biochemical abnormality led to the x-ray being taken?
c What is the underlying metabolic disorder?
d Suggest two possible causes for his abdominal pain.

570 This patient's haemoglobin is 18g/dl. White cell and platelet counts are normal. Isotope red cell mass study shows normal plasma volume and an absolute increase in red cell mass. A non-smoker, she is moderately breathless on exertion but has no other respiratory symptoms. She has a tendency to fall asleep during the day.

a What unusual cause of the haematological findings is suggested by her appearances?

b What name is given to the disorder?

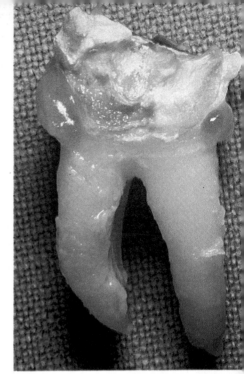

571

571 and 572

a What condition links these two pictures?

b What is the most common causal agent?

c Which structural cardiac abnormality is generally said *not* to predispose to this condition?

572

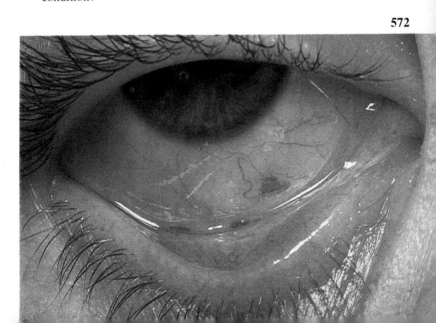

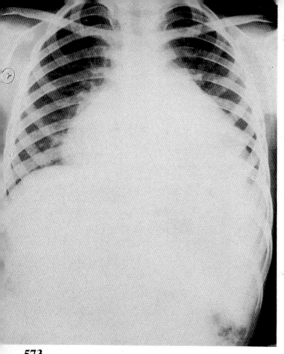

573

573 This patient with rheumatoid arthritis complains of gradually increasing tiredness, breathlessness and ankle swelling. There is no history of valvular heart disease.
a What is the principal radiological abnormality?
b What is the likely diagnosis?
c List the clinical features which you might elicit on examination of the cardiovascular system.

574

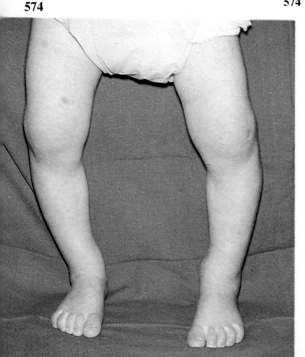

574 a What radiological abnormalities are likely to be present in this child?
b What is the diagnosis?

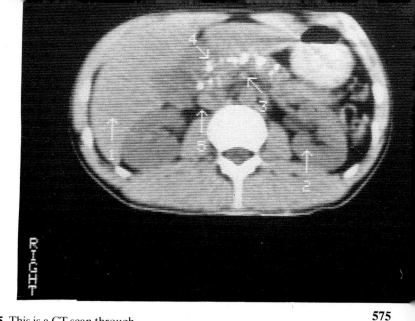

575 This is a CT scan through
the pancreas of a thirty
year old male. He is a
chronic alcoholic and has
recurrent abdominal pain.
   a Name the structures
      labelled 1-5 and
      indicate the
      abnormalities present.
   b What is the likely
      diagnosis?

576 This patient has
thyrotoxicosis. In
addition to symptoms of
hyperthyroidism, she
complains of difficulty in
swallowing.
List three clinical signs
which may suggest
retrosternal extension of
her goitre.

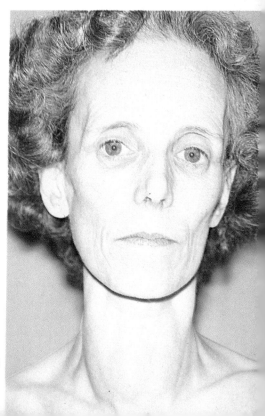

576

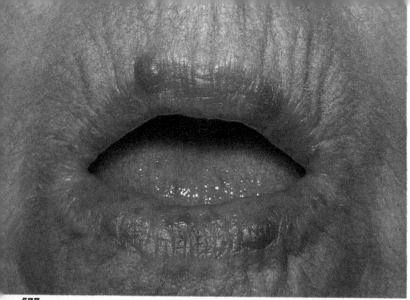

577

577 and 578 This person's only complaint is of recurrent epistaxis.
  a What is the diagnosis?
  b What is the most likely cause of the radiological appearance?
  c What other facial sign may be seen in this condition?

578

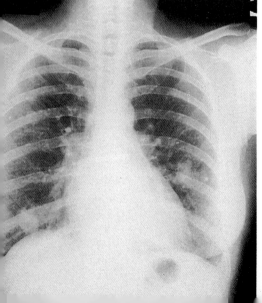

579 a What abnormality of this neonate's ear is seen?

b With which maternal disorder is this typically associated?

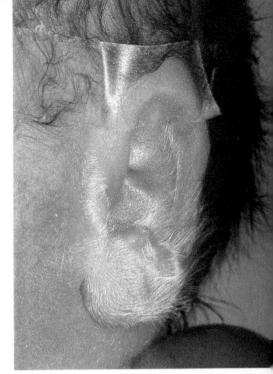

580 This patient was treated five years ago with venesection and ^{32}phosphorus for polycythaemia rubra vera. She now presents with anaemia of 8.9g/dl, white cell count of 3.5 x 10^9/1 and platelets 110 x 10^9/1.

a What abnormality does this film demonstrate and what diagnosis is likely?

b What would bone marrow aspiration reveal?

c What abnormality is likely to be found on clinical examination?

579

580

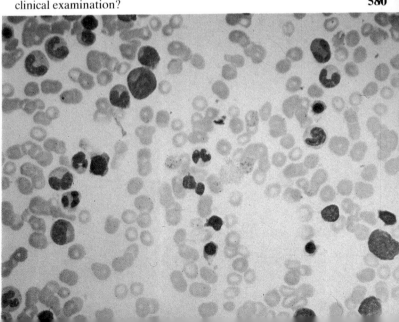

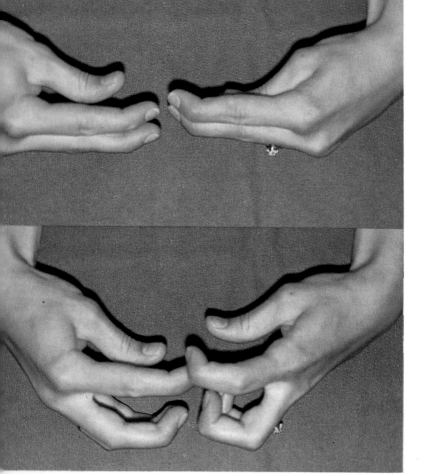

581 and 582 This patient was asked to oppose her thumbs, as shown in the first picture. She was then asked to open all her fingers as quickly as possible. The second picture was taken two seconds after she first began to open her fingers.

a What phenomenon is demonstrated?

b How is this phenomenon's passive form most simply demonstrated?

c Which disorders does this typify?

ANSWERS

The answers given below are necessarily brief as the aim of the series is to stimulate self-learning through further reading.

389 and 390
- a i) Right Horner's syndrome.
  - ii) Right twelfth cranial nerve palsy.
- b i) Jugular foramen lesions (ie at or outside the foramen). eg meningioma, neurofibroma, glomus jugulare tumour.
  - ii) Syringomyelia/syringobulbia.
  - iii) Brainstem vascular disease — sympathetic fibres lie dorsolaterally, twelfth nerve nucleus dorsomedially. Combination of Horner's and twelfth nerve palsy can occur, but implies extensive infarction of one half of the medulla.

391 and 392
- a Leprosy.
- b Resorption of the phalanges of third to fifth toes, and of fourth metacarpal of both feet.
- c No. The lepromin test is of value in classifying the type of disease but is of no diagnostic value.
- d There is no animal reservoir. Patients with lepromatous leprosy are the probable source of infection.

393 a A — posterior prolapse of the mitral valve leaflets in systole.
B — echoes from redundant posterior mitral valve tissue in diastole (these echoes should not be confused with calcification or prolapsing left atrial tumour).
- b Mitral valve prolapse ('floppy' mitral valve).
- c Systolic click (or clicks) followed by an apical crescendo-decrescendo late systolic murmur.
(Occasionally, a pansystolic murmur, without systolic click, is present).

394 a Obesity, gynaecomastia, small external genitalia.
- b Klinefelter's syndrome.

395 Background diabetic retinopathy with microaneurysms and small haemorrhages.

396 a Bifid P in VI; complete right bundle branch block; right axis deviation; Q waves VI-4; ST depression II, III, AVF; T inversion VI-5; a single ventricular extrasystole.

    b Yes. Bifascicular block (Right bundle branch block and left posterior hemiblock) has the same significance as left bundle branch block.

    c Anteroseptal myocardial infarction. The ST depression in the inferior leads may be due to digoxin administration.

397 a Extensive bilateral nodular opacities particularly in the upper and mid zones; "egg-shell" calcification of hilar lymph nodes.

    b Silicosis.

    c i) No.

        ii) Yes.

398 a Necrobiosis lipoidica.

    b Diabetes mellitus.

    c There is no consistent relationship between severity of necrobiosis and duration or adequacy of glycaemic control of diabetes. Necrobiosis may precede the development of glucose intolerance.

399 a Elephantiasis.

    b The filarial worm, Wuchereria bancrofti.
       (May occasionally follow tuberculous lymphadenitis).

    c Adult worms might be seen. Lymph node biopsy further compromises lymphatic drainage, however, and should not be carried out.

400 a Pharyngeal pouch.

    b Recurrent aspiration of food material may lead to

        i) Pneumonia (typically right lower lobe).

        ii) Bronchiectasis.

        iii) Lung abscess.

    c Perforation, with mediastinitis.

401 a i)   Gynaecomastia.

        ii)   Undue bruising at venepuncture sites.

    b Alcoholic liver disease.
       (The tattoo raises the possibility of chronic hepatitis following Hepatitis B infection).

402 Homogentisate (patient has alkaptonuria; the illustration shows disc calcification of ochronosis).

403 a 'Bull neck'; enlarged cervical nodes.

    b Chronic lymphatic leukaemia.

    c Corticosteroids. (Because of autoimmune haemolysis.)

404 a Hypoglycaemia.

    b i)   Change to highly purified insulin injections.

        ii)   Rotation of sites of insulin injections.

405 and 406

    a i)   Basal ganglia calcification.

        ii)   Short 4th and 5th metacarpals.

b Pseudohypoparathyroidism.
c i) Low serum calcium, high serum phosphate.
   ii) Normal or increased serum parathormone level.
   iii) Subnormal response of urinary cyclic AMP following intravenous
        injection of parathyroid extract.

407 a Tuberculous peritonitis.
b i) Ziehl-Nielsen stain of ascitic fluid.
  ii) Cultures for T.B.
  iii) Mantoux.
  iv) Peritoneal biopsy.

408 a Macular choroiditis.
b Toxoplasmosis.
c He may have a cerebral toxoplasma abscess.
d Acquired immune deficiency syndrome.

409 a Coeliac disease. (Crohn's disease is a less likely possibility).
b i) HLA — B8.
  ii) HLA — DW3.

410 a Trousseau's sign.
b Indicates latent tetany.
c i) Hypocalcaemia.
  ii) Hypokalaemia.
  iii) Hypomagnesaemia.
  iv) Metabolic or respiratory alkalosis.

411 a Exophthalmos, lid retraction, periorbital oedema, mild cheimosis
b Graves' ophthalmopathy (endocrine exophthalmos).
c i) Corneal ulceration.
  ii) Extraocular muscle paresis (may be complete).
  iii) Papilloedema, optic neuritis.
d i) Mild — symptomatic — methylcellulose drops.
  ii) Lid retraction — guanethidine eye drops.
  iii) Surgical — tarsorrhaphy.
              — surgical decompression.
  iv) Corticosteroids, immunosuppressive drugs, irradiation in
      progressive/malignant exophthalmos.

412 a External fistula.
b Crohn's disease.
c Acute ileitis.

413 a Lid lag.
b Thyrotoxicosis.
c i) Lid retraction, globe lag.
  ii) Exophthalmos, proptosis, conjunctival oedema,
      ophthalmoplegia.
  iii) Tremor of lightly closed lids.

414 a Autoimmune thrombocytopaenic purpura.
  b Normal or increased numbers of megakaryocytes of normal morphology.
  c Drug induced thrombocytopaenia; post-infective thrombocytopaenia; systemic lupus erythematosus with bone-marrow failure; disseminated intravascular coagulation; lymphoma.

415 a Generalised amyloidosis.
  b Rectal, gingival, or renal biopsy.

416 These include,
  i) Bronchial carcinoma (occasionally, secondary malignancies).
  ii) Chronic suppuration — bronchiectasis, empyema, abscess.
  iii) Some causes of interstitial lung disease: especially fibrosing alveolitis (idiopathic), asbestosis.
  iv) Benign pleural fibroma.

417 a No.
  b Lung volumes may be normal or there may be reduction of vital capacity and total lung capacity. Transfer factor is normal.

418 a Tuberous xanthomata.
  b Type IIa or III hyperlipidaemia.
  c Fasting lipoproteins.
  d Low cholesterol diet.
  Identification and, if present, treatment of diabetes mellitus or hypothyroidism. Clofibrate, cholestyramine, probucol, bezafibrate.

419 a Epstein-Barr virus, causing infectious mononucleosis.
  b Chronic lymphocytic leukaemia; cytomegalovirus infection.
  c Yes, if there is no previous history of penicillin sensitivity.

420 a Chronic left subdural haematoma. (The clot is hypodense compared with brain and therefore is more than three weeks old.)
  b Head injury which may be relatively minor and therefore easily forgotten; cerebral atrophy which renders the emissary veins more susceptible to rupture.

421 and 422
  a Sclerosis and ankylosis of the sacroiliac joints.
  b A scaling rash.
  c Psoriatic arthropathy.
  d Approximately one in three.

423 a Lipohypertrophy ("insulin tumours").
  b The hypertrophy can be explained by the known action of insulin on the synthesis of lipids by fat cells.
  c Vary site of insulin injections and avoid these sites of hypertrophy.

424 a Acromegaly.
   b i) Plasma growth hormone excess and non-suppression during oral glucose tolerance test.
      ii) Confirm presence of pituitary adenoma — skull x-ray ± computed tomography of pituitary fossa.

425 and 426
   a Widespread periostitis.
   b Rhagades.
   c Congenital syphilis.

427 a Burr cells, anisocytosis.
   b i) Reduced erythropoietin secretion.
      ii) Impaired utilisation of iron.
      iii) Increased haemolysis.
      iv) Increased blood loss, eg from the gastrointestinal tract or during haemodialysis.
      v) Folate deficiency which may be nutritional deficiency or loss during dialysis.

428 a Otitis externa.
   b Pseudomonas aeruginosa and Proteus mirabilis.
   c Yes; regular application of aluminium acetate in 2.5% acetic acid ear drops prior to and during saturation diving dramatically reduces the incidence of this disease.

429 a i) Short stature (shortening of the lower half of the body in particular).
      ii) Genu valgum.
   b i) Hypophosphataemia.
      ii) Phosphaturia.
      iii) Raised alkaline phosphatase in more severe cases in excess of the normally high childhood levels.
      iv) Hydroxyprolinuria.
      Parathormone levels vary; aminoaciduria and glycosuria are occasionally found.
   c Condition is transmitted as x-linked dominant. Risk is therefore 100%.

430 a Livedo reticularis.
   b i) Systemic lupus erythematosus (false positive TPHA).
      ii) Syphilis.

431 and 432
   a i) Distended left external jugular vein.
      ii) Swelling and discolouration.
   b i) Subclavian venous obstruction.
      (The external jugular is a tributary of the subclavian vein: it is not necessary to postulate brachiocephalic (innominate) venous obstruction).

ii) Bronchogenic carcinoma. He has nicotine staining on the fingers of his right hand, and appears to have finger clubbing. There is a radiotherapy marker on the right chest. The lesion on his left forearm is a surgical scar (from excision of tattoo) and is not infected.

433 and 434
    a Hydrocortisone, fludrocortisone.
    b Addison's disease.

435 a Deviation to the right; early wasting.
      b No.
      c Medial medullary syndrome. Infarction of the medial medulla involving the hypoglossal nerve, medial lemniscus, and medullary pyramid.

436 a Reflex sympathetic dystrophy — the shoulder-hand syndrome.
      b Trauma, hemiplegia, and cervical spondylosis are associated but in some cases there may be no identifiable cause.
      c Physiotherapy is the mainstay of treatment; short courses of oral corticosteroids or local injection of corticosteroids have also proved beneficial.

437 a i)   Tonsillar enlargement.
         ii)   Tonsillar exudate.
         iii) Palatal petechiae.
      b Infectious mononucleosis (glandular fever).

438 a Erythema nodosum.
      b i)   Sulphonamides.
         ii)   Oral contraceptives.

439 a Turner's syndrome.
      b 45XO, XX/XO (Turner mosaic) or 46XX (Noonan's).
      c Coarctation of the aorta. Others include: bicuspid aortic valve, aortic stenosis, atrial septal defect, pulmonary stenosis (especially in Noonan's).

440 a White nails (the colour change here is in the nail bed: this is not true leukonychia where the nail plate is white).
      b Hepatic cirrhosis (hypoalbuminaemia need not be present).

441 a Tuberculosis (lupus vulgaris).
      b Pressure under a glass slide may reveal characteristic "apple jelly" nodules.

442 i)   Leprosy.
       ii)   Syphilis.

443, 444 and 445
    a Hand, foot and mouth disease.
    b Coxsackie A 16.

446 a Tethering and fibrosis of the right inferior rectus muscle.
    b The intraocular pressure may rise on attempted upward gaze.

447 a Thrombosis of the central retinal vein.
    b Hypertension; arteriosclerosis; diabetes mellitus; polycythaemia rubra vera; hyperviscosity syndromes.

448 Possibilities include
    i) Cutaneous leishmaniasis: leishmaniasis recidiva.
    ii) Cutaneous tuberculosis.
    iii) Tertiary syphilis.

449 a Recurrent burning pain in the feet, with redness and increased temperature, provoked by local heat or increase in ambient temperature, exercise (walking, running) or standing (that is, factors which normally induce peripheral vasodilatation).
    b i) Systemic lupus erythematosus.
      ii) Hypertension.
      iii) Polycythaemia rubra vera.
      iv) Other myeloproliferative disorders.
      v) Idiopathic.

450 a Rose spot of typhoid.
    b Yes.
    c Splenomegaly and hepatomegaly may occur. Abdominal distension and tenderness are usually present. Peritonism may occur with perforation.

451 a No. These are venereal warts, not secondary syphilis.
    b They include podophyllin, trichloracetic acid, and electro-cautery.

452 a Left renal vein thrombosis.
    b Loss of antithrombin III through the glomeruli in the nephrotic syndrome.
    c Amyloidosis secondary to osteomyelitis.

453 Toxoplasmosis, toxocariasis, cytomegalovirus, tuberculosis, syphilis, rubella.

454 and 455
    a Pellagra (nicotinic acid deficiency).
    b Carcinoid syndrome.
    c Estimation of urinary 5-hydroxy indole acetic acid.

456 a Aphthous ulcers.
    b Behçet's disease.

c i) Central (or branch) retinal venous occlusion.
  ii) Dural venous thrombosis (eg superior sagittal sinus thrombosis).
  iii) Superior or inferior vena caval obstruction.
    (Any vein or venous system may, however, be affected).

457 a Congenital dislocation of the hip (with false acetabulum).
  b Yes; it should be detected at birth by routine clinical examination.

458 a Enlarged accessory and great auricular nerves.
  b i) Leprosy.
   ii) Amyloidosis.
   iii) Neurofibromatosis.
   iv) Hypertrophic peripheral neuropathy (Dejerine-Sottas disease).
   v) Refsum's disease.

459 a Hypopyon (pus in the anterior chamber).
  b Crohn's disease; ulcerative colitis; sarcoidosis; Behçet's disease;
    tuberculosis.

460 a Atrial fibrillation.
  b i) Ischaemic heart disease.
   ii) Rheumatic heart disease.
   iii) Thyrotoxicosis.
   iv) Acute infections.
   v) Hypertension.
   vi) Constrictive pericarditis.
   Less common causes include lone atrial fibrillation; atrial septal
   defect; acute pericarditis; cardiomyopathy; Wolff-Parkinson-White
   syndrome; thoracic surgery.

461 a There is increased lucency of the left lower lobe of lung; acquired
    hypoplastic emphysema of childhood (McLeod's syndrome).
  b It is thought to be secondary to bronchiolitis during childhood.
  c There is a marked reduction in breath sounds over the affected area.

462 a Gilbert's disease.
  b Liver histology is normal.
  c i) Compensated haemolysis (ie in which reduced red cell survival is
     offset by increased red cell production).
   ii) 'Shunt' hyperbilirubinaemia, (in which there is abnormal
     haemoglobin destruction in marrow red cell precursors. Survival
     of peripheral red cells is typically normal).
     Crigler Najaar syndrome (congenital glucuronyl transferase
     deficiency), type II (milder, autosomal dominant form) is an
     outside possibility.

463 a Otitis media.
  b Streptococcus pneumoniae; Haemophilus influenzae; Staphylococcus
  pyogenes; Pseudomonas; Proteus.

464 a No. The lesion is compressing the calcarine cortex.
     b Meningioma.

465 a Calcified cysts in the calf muscles.
     b Cerebral cysticercosis (cysts are not usually seen on plain skull x-ray).
     c Praziquantel.

466 a Migratory thrombophlebitis.
     b Pancreatic tumour.

467 a Soft tissue mass arising in left hypochondrium, displacing large bowel: appearance suggests massive splenomegaly.
      Causes include:
     b i)   Chronic myeloid leukaemia.
        ii) Myelofibrosis.
        iii) Kala-azar.
        iv) Gaucher's disease.
        v)   Malaria.
        vi) Tropical splenomegaly syndrome.

468 a Campbell de Morgan spots (cherry angiomas).
     b They are a normal feature (although increased numbers have been described in diabetes mellitus).

469 a Psoriasis (arthritis mutilans).
     b Asymmetrical distal interphalangeal arthropathy; seronegative polyarthropathy resembling rheumatoid arthritis; asymmetric oligoarthritis; ankylosing spondylitis; gout.
     c No. They may cause a severe exfoliative dermatitis.

470 a Osteomyelitis.
     b Salmonella species.

471 a Disciform degeneration of the macula.
     b Photocoagulation may occasionaly be beneficial if the fovea is not directly involved.
     c None.

472 a Orf.
     b Bacterial superinfection.
      Erythema multiforme.

473 a Meningococcal septicaemia.
     b Intravenous benzylpenicillin.
     c Markedly elevated cortisol.

474 a Chronic venous insufficiency with varicose veins and varicose eczema.
     b i)   Antithrombin III deficiency.
       ii) Protein C deficiency.

475 and 476
  a Chronic tophaceous gout.
  b Acute gout may be precipitated.
  c They are the source of colchicine, a useful drug in the treatment of acute gout.

477 a Dermographism.
  b Histamine.

478 a Chancre (primary syphilis).
  b Microscopy of expressed serum using dark-ground illumination.

479 a i) Left ptosis.
  ii) Constricted left pupil.
  b Left Horner's syndrome.

480 a i) Flame-shaped and blot haemorrhages.
  ii) Hard exudates, partial macular star.
  iii) Soft exudates (cotton wool spots).
  iv) Papilloedema.
  v) Arteriovenous 'nipping' and angulation.
  vi) Arteriolar irregularity in calibre and silver wiring.
  b Hypertension (accelerated).

481 and 482
  Reticulohistiocytosis.

483 None. A geographical tongue is shown.

484 a Malignant melanoma.
  b Choroid.
  c i) Direct invasion and destruction of retinal tissue (and ultimately of adjacent structures).
  ii) Retinal detachment.
  iii) Glaucoma.

485 a Varicosity of superficial abdominal veins.
  b Obstruction of inferior vena cava.

486 a Single transverse palmar crease (simian crease).
  b Down's syndrome (Trisomy 21).
  c Clinodactyly (incurving of the fifth finger).

487 and 488
  a Bruising in the flank/groin.
  b Anterior erosion of lumbar vertebral bodies.
  c Abdominal aortic aneurysm.

489 a Hutchinson's lentigo (lentigo maligna melanoma — a chronic radially spreading melanoma).
  b Development of a vertically invasive nodule of malignant melanoma.

490   i)   Lichen sclerosus.
          ii) Morphoea (localised scleroderma).

491 a Sinus tachycardia; S_I, Q_{III}, T_{III} pattern.
       b Pulmonary thromboembolism.
       c Intravenous heparin or streptokinase.

492 and 493
     a i)   Increased anteroposterior diameter.
          ii) Finger clubbing.
     b Cystic fibrosis.
     c i)   Pancreatic enzyme supplement ($\pm$histamine$_2$ receptor
             antagonist).
          ii) Fat-soluble vitamin supplements.

494 a Target lesions.
       b Erythema multiforme.
       c Haemoglobinuria (secondary to intravascular haemolysis).
       d Mycoplasma pneumonia.
       e Serum cold agglutinins, mycoplasma complement fixation test.

495 a Right upper lobe consolidation with cavitation.
       b i)   Tuberculosis.
          ii) Staphylococcus aureus.
       c i)   Infective consolidation with abscess formation (may be primary
             pneumonia, or secondary to proximal bronchial obstruction/
             stenosis, or pulmonary infarction).
             Other organisms include klebsiella, pseudomonas, proteus,
             anaerobic bacteria, fungi (aspergillus, histoplasmosis,
             coccidioidomycosis).
          ii) Cavitating primary (squamous) or secondary (squamous,
             sarcomata) neoplasm.
          iii) Pulmonary infarction (without infection).
          iv) Infective consolidation with pre-existing apical bullae.

496 and 497
     a Rheumatoid arthritis (RA).
     b Pleural fluid associated with RA is typically an exudate. It contains
        high protein, low glucose, and numerous lymphocytes
     c Swan neck deformity is due to increased tension in the intrinsic
        muscles. This is usually due to synovial thickening or anterior
        subluxation of the metacarpophalangeal joints. Laxity or destruction
        of the volar plate of the proximal interphalangeal joint allows the
        intrinsic muscles to hyperextend the proximal interphalangeal joint
        and flex the metacarpophalangeal joint, with the distal
        interphalangeal joint flexed by the profundus tendon.

498 a Vitreous haemorrhage.
       b Proliferative retinopathy.
       c Permanent visual loss; glaucoma; fibrosis with traction retinal
        detachment.

499 a Superficial spreading malignant melanoma.
    b The depth of invasion, since survival is inversely proportional to this.

500 a i)   Loss of red reflex, with central mature cataract.
      ii)   Irregular pupil with posterior synechiae.
      iii) Rubeosis iridis.
      iv) Hyphaema.
      v)   Astigmatic cornea.
    b Central retinal venous thrombosis.

501 The right submammary scar is coincidental.
    a Cushingoid facies — mooned face, plethora, truncal obesity, muscle wasting especially of thighs.
    b Cushing's syndrome.
    c i)   Iatrogenic.
      ii)   Adrenal tumour (adenoma or carcinoma) most likely in this age group.
      iii) Pituitary-driven (not common in this age group).

502 a Central neck swelling.
    b Simple goitre. Patient does not show facial features of thyrotoxicosis or myxoedema.
    c i)   Serum thyroid hormone concentration — Thyroxine (T4) and Tri-iodothyronine (T3).
      ii)   Serum thyroid stimulating hormone.
      iii) Thyroid antibodies.
      iv) Thyroid scan (isotopic).
      v)   (Percutaneous fine needle biopsy with cytology).

503 a Swelling of the optic nerve head (papillitis).
    b Retrobulbar neuritis.
    c Marcus Gunn pupil.

504 a Ischaemia.
      ('Saddle' thromboembolic obstruction of the aortic bifurcation).
    b i)   Heparinisation.
      ii)   Arterial embolectomy.
      iii) Pain relief.

505 a Lymphangitis carcinomatosa (lymphatic carcinomatosis) (linear shadows radiating from the hila).
    b i)   Prominent hila.
      ii)   Absent right breast shadow.
              — breast carcinoma with secondary mediastinal involvement and pulmonary lymphatic obstruction or infiltration.

506 a Upper mediastinal opacity, behind the trachea.
    b i)   Neural tumour (from intercostal nerve, sympathetic chain) e.g. neurofibroma, ganglioneuroma.

ii) Paravertebral mass (e.g. tuberculous abscess).
iii) Bronchogenic cyst.

507 a Evidence of previous intravenous drug administration ('mainlining').
b Intravenous administration of naloxone.

508 a Episcleritis.
b These include rheumatoid arthritis, tuberculosis, streptococcal infections.

509 a Gangrene of the first toes.
b Surgical treatment of ingrowing toenails.

510 a Secondary bacterial infection (Impetigo).
b i) Staphylococcus pyogenes.
   ii) Streptococcus pyogenes.

511 i) Systemic lupus erythematosus.
ii) Scleroderma.

512 a Herpes gestationis.
b There is no relation to herpes viruses. Circulating complement-fixing factor and anti-basement membrane Immunoglobulins G have been demonstrated.
c Yes, almost certainly.

513 a Retinitis pigmentosa.
b i) "Night blindness" — unusually poor visual acuity in poor lighting conditions (eg. at night).
   ii) In this case since there are also macular changes the patient is also likely to complain of loss of daytime visual acuity, and may be aware of a defect in central vision.

514 a Cerebellopontine angle lesion (neuroma of the VIIth nerve more likely than acoustic neuroma in the presence of VIIth nerve palsy).
b i) Tinnitus, hearing loss are not features of Bell's palsy (although hyperacusis may be).
   ii) Absent corneal reflex implies loss of corneal sensation (Vth nerve). Eye lid closure may be impaired in isolated VIIth nerve palsy, but corneal sensation and consensual closure of the other eyelid are preserved.

515 a Peutz-Jegher syndrome.
b Hamartomatous intestinal polyposis.
c Risk is 1 in 2. Inheritance is autosomal dominant.

516 and 517
a i) Hypoplasia (and splitting of the right nail).
   ii) Absent patella.
b Nail — patella syndrome.
c Proteinuria (found in about forty per cent).

518 a i) Left sided emphysema (not pneumothorax).
   ii) Mediastinal shift to left.
   b Ball-valve obstruction of left main bronchus, secondary to inhalation of a foreign body (in this case, a peanut).

519 a Anisopoikilocytosis with hypochromic microcytic erythrocytes, target cells and normoblasts.
   b Beta-thalassaemia major.
   c i) Regular iron chelation with desferrioxamine which may be given by subcutaneous infusion.
   ii) Folic acid supplements.
   iii) Ascorbic acid supplements, which enhance iron excretion by desferrioxamine.

520 a Janeway lesions.
   b Infective endocarditis.

521 a Vitiligo.
   b i) Cosmetic cover.
   ii) Oral psoralen with sunlight or artificial ultraviolet light.
   iii) Topical fluorinated corticosteroids.
   iv) If there is residual hyperpigmentation in the presence of extensive depigmentation, a bleaching cream (eg. hydroquinone) may be used.

522 a Extensive anterior myocardial infarction.
   b i) Prophylaxis against venous thrombosis.
   ii) Treatment of established venous thrombosis with or without pulmonary thromboembolism.
   iii) Treatment of systemic thromboembolism resulting from mural thrombus.

523 a Distension of the external jugular vein.
   b None. i) in this case, the vein is compressed between platysma and sternomastoid on neck turning.
   ii) jugular venous pressure may be raised without elevated right atrial pressures eg. in superior vena caval obstruction.

524 a Bouchard's (proximal interphalangeal) and Heberden's nodes (distal interphalangeal).
   b Primary osteoarthrosis.
   c Distal interphalangeal; proximal interphalangeal; first carpometacarpal; occasionally, metacarpophalangeal.

525 a Scleromalacia.
   b Rheumatoid arthritis.

526 i) Oval macrocytosis.
   ii) Polymorph nuclear hypersegmentation.
   iii) Moderate neutropenia, lymphopenia, thrombocytopenia.

iv) Reticulocyte count/degree of polychromasia inappropriately low for degree of anaemia.
v) Evidence of red cell fragmentation.
vi) Anisopoikilocytosis.
vii) Leucoerythroblastic picture (extramedullary haemopoiesis).

527 a Pericardial (springwater cyst).
  b i) Pericardial diverticulum.
    ii) Hernia through the foramen of Morgagni.
    Pericardial fat pads are of low radiodensity and triangular in shape and should not be confused with pericardial cysts.

528 a Myxoedema 'coma'.
  b i) Thyroid hormone deficiency.
    ii) Cortisol deficiency.
    iii) Hypoglycaemia.
    iv) Hypercapnia.
    v) Hyponatraemia.
    vi) Hypoxia.
    vii) Features of coincidental renal or hepatic failure.

529 a Acute paronychia.
  b Staphylococcus aureus.
  c Incision (at the site of pointing: seen as a 'head' just proximal to the nailbed) using a fine pointed scalpel. Antibiotic is unnecessary.

530 a There is a large low-density area in the right fronto-parietal region which represents infarction in the territory of the right middle cerebral artery.
  b Left hemiplegia, homonymous hemianopia and hemianaesthesia.
  c There may be conjugate deviation to the right due to damage to the right frontal region responsible for voluntary gaze.

531 a Left third cranial nerve palsy due to a posterior communicating aneurysm which has ruptured causing a sub-arachnoid haemorrhage.
  b Diplopia is not a feature of Horner's syndrome.
  c Cerebral CT scan if available. Lumbar puncture will be required if the CT scan is negative or unavailable.

532 a Thymectomy through a combined median sternotomy and cervical approach. Myasthenia gravis.
  b He may have a thymoma (more likely in view of age of onset and sex) or thymitis.
  c Aminoglycosides.

533 a Papilloedema, hard and soft exudates ('cotton wool spots'), subhyaloid and nerve-fibre layer haemorrhages, and arteriolar irregularity.
  b Accelerated hypertension.

534 a Idiopathic Raynaud's phenomenon.
    b There is a very low risk and there are usually no long term sequelae apart from its nuisance value.
    c Beta blockers; ergot derivatives; methysergide; (tobacco).

535 a Molluscum contagiosum.
    b No.

536 a Rickets (Vitamin D deficiency).
    b i) Similar bony expansion at the wrists.
      ii) Pectus carinatum (pigeon chest).
      iii) 'Rickety rosary' — expansion of the costochondral junctions.
      iv) Genu valgum (or varum).
      v) Skull abnormalities — softening (craniotabes), frontal bossing.

537 a Dupuytren's contracture.
    b Porphyria cutanea tarda (PCT).
    c It is not inherited. PCT is an acquired condition, usually due to alcoholic liver disease.
    d i) Avoidance of alcohol.
      ii) Regular venesection.

538 a Hydatid cyst. (His coughing bout represented intra-bronchial rupture of another cyst.)
    b Ingestion of the tapeworm echinococcus granulosus after handling infected dogs (the usual definitive host) or ingestion of contaminated food or water.
    c Acute anaphylaxis.

539 a Corneal opacification ('cloudy cornea').
    b Hurler's syndrome.
    c Heparan sulphate and dermatan sulphate.

540 a Thyroid carcinoma.
    b A 'cold' spot.

541 a Acute gout.
    b Septic arthritis.
    c Aspiration of the affected joint.

542 a Mitral stenosis.
    b i) Increasingly long diastolic murmur.
      ii) Approximation of second sound and opening snap.
      iii) Opening snap and diastolic murmur may soften and disappear.
      iv) Loud pulmonary second sound and pulmonary diastolic murmur with development of pulmonary hypertension.
    c Diastolic pressure gradient across the mitral valve (measured at cardiac catheterisation).

543 a Widespread small nodular opacities of calcific density. (Miliary calcification).
   b i) Tuberculosis.
   ii) Chickenpox.
   iii) Histoplasmosis.
   (In each case appearance is that of healed pneumonia).

544 a Spider telangiectasia (spider naevus).
   b i) Normal finding.
   ii) Liver disease.
   iii) Pregnancy.

545 a Neurofibromatosis.
   b Phaeochromocytoma (occurs in approximately 1% of patients with neurofibromatosis).
   c Autosomal dominant.

546 a Onycholysis.
   b i) Idiopathic ($\pm$ minor trauma $\pm$ frequent immersion in water).
   ii) Dermatological disorders — psoriasis, eczema.
   iii) Fungal infection (tinea unguium).
   iv) General medical, including hypo- and hyperthyroidism, peripheral circulatory disorders.
   v) Drugs — eg. tetracyclines, in association with photosensitivity.

547 Malunited forearm fracture.

548 a Congenital ptosis.
   b Amblyopia may develop if unilateral ptosis obscures the visual axis.

549 and 550
   a i) Right hilar enlargement.
   ii) Opacity over anterior end of 5th rib.
   b Primary tuberculosis (The lumps on the legs suggest erythema nodosum).

551 a Fracture of mid shaft of humerus.
   b Radial.
   c i) motor — loss of action of brachioradialis, supinator, all forearm extensors. (triceps will be spared)
   ii) sensory — small area of sensory loss in the web between thumb and forefinger.

552 a i) Shortening of the PR interval.
   ii) Widening of the QRS complex.
   iii) Slurring of the R upstroke, resulting in a delta wave.
   b Wolff-Parkinson-White syndrome, type A.
   c His fits may be due to cerebral anoxia resulting from a tachyarrhythmia as a consequence of WPW syndrome.

553 a Ringworm: tinea corporis.
  b All known dermatophytes can cause this (i.e. microsporum, trichophyton and epidermophyton species).
  c Griseofulvin.

554 a Corneal arcus.
  b Raised low density lipoprotein (LDL) concentration.
  c Age.

555 a Benign intracranial hypertension.
  b Oral contraceptives, chronic corticosteroid administration, acute steroid withdrawal, tetracyclines, vitamin D

556 Inclusion dermoid.

557 a Gas under the right hemidiaphragm.
  b Perforated viscus (in this case, perforated duodenal ulcer is most likely).

558 and 559
  a Geniculate zoster (Ramsay-Hunt syndrome).
  b Vth, VIIIth and IXth nerve involvement may occur.
  c She has about a 50% chance of full recovery.

560 a A Gross ascites.
    B Small bowel seen in transverse section.
    C Normal mesentery.
  b Loops of small bowel and mesentery float and are separated by free fluid.

561 and 562
  a Tuberculous pleural effusion, with a positive Mantoux test.
  b Very slight. Pleural biopsy is much more likely to be diagnostic.

563 a Paget's disease.
  b Bone conduction heard louder than air conduction. (In Paget's disease, deafness is more commonly secondary to ossicular involvement than to foraminal compression and sensorineural loss).

564 a Yellow discolouration.
  b Lymphoedema (secondary to lymphatic atresia or functional lymphatic insufficiency) — she has the 'yellow nail syndrome'.

565 a Facioscapulohumeral muscular dystrophy.
  b Autosomal dominant inheritance (rarely it may be recessive).
  c No. Pelvic involvement is rarely significant.

566 a Menisceal calcification.
  b Pseudogout.
  c Calcium pyrophosphate crystals.

567 a Pupillary irregularity due to posterior synechiae.
    b Anterior uveitis.
    c These include Crohn's disease, ulcerative colitis. Reiter's disease may also present in this way.

568 a Koebner phenomenon.
    b i) Skin injury.
      ii) Sunburn or local heat, eg in association with erythema ab igne.
      iii) Vaccination scars.
      iv) At sites of other coexistent skin eruptions.
    c i) Psoriasis.
      ii) Lichen planus.
      iii) Acute eczema.
      iv) Warts (especially plane warts).

569 a Multiple lucencies — 'pepperpot' skull.
    b Hypercalcaemia.
    c Hyperparathyroidism.
    d i) Acute peptic ulcer.
      ii) Acute pancreatitis.

570 a Chronic hypoxia secondary to hypoventilation.
    b 'Pickwickian' syndrome.

571 and 572
    a Infective endocarditis.
    b Streptococcus viridans.
    c i) Ostium secundum atrial septal defect.
      ii) Severe mitral stenosis, where turbulence is restricted by diminished blood flow through the valve, is also said not to predispose.

573 a Massive cardiomegaly.
    b Pericardial effusion.
    c i) Signs of low cardiac output — narrow pulse pressure, tachycardia, peripheral vasoconstriction and cyanosis.
      ii) Pulsus paradoxus.
      iii) Raised jugular venous pressure, unaffected by or paradoxically rising with inspiration (Kussmaul's sign).
      iv) Impalpable apex beat (not necessarily).
      v) Increased area of cardiac dullness.
      vi) Heart sounds diminished in intensity (but may be normal). Added sounds (eg third, fourth sounds) or pericardial rub unlikely.
      vii) Ankle, sacral oedema, ascites. Basal lung crackles.
      viii) Signs of consolidation at left lung base (increased vocal fremitus, bronchial breath sounds, bronchophony, whispering pectoriloquy) occasionally heard — Ewart's sign (probably secondary to left lower lobe compression).

574 a The epiphyseal growth plate will be widened and the metaphysis cupped and ragged.
  b Rickets.

575 a 1 Right lower lobe of liver.
    2 Left kidney.
    3 Superior mesenteric artery.
    4 Pancreas: slightly enlarged with multiple areas of calcification in the head and body.
    5 Inferior vena cava.
  b Recurrent acute pancreatitis.

576 i) Displacement of the suprasternal portion of the trachea.
    ii) Stridor.
    iii) Arm raising test — if significant retrosternal extension is present, raising the arms above the head (thereby reducing the size of the thoracic inlet) may lead to facial congestion and respiratory distress ($\pm$ stridor) — Pemberton's sign.

577 and 578
  a Hereditary haemorrhagic telangiectasia.
  b Pulmonary arteriovenous fistulae.
  c Central cyanosis if there is a significant right to left shunt.

579 a Hairy ear.
  b Diabetes mellitus.

580 a Leucoerythroblastic reaction; myelofibrosis (myelosclerosis).
  b It is likely to show nothing as attempts at marrow aspiration are usually unsuccessful in myelofibrosis.
  c Massive splenomegaly and, to a lesser extent, hepatomegaly are almost always present.

581 and 582
  a Active myotonia.
  b By percussion of the thenar eminence, forearm extensor tendons or achilles tendon. Sustained contraction of the appropriate muscle groups results.
  c Myotonic dystrophies — myotonic dystrophy, myotonia congenita (Thomsen's disease).

INDEX